THE *REAL* RULES FOR BEING THE WOMAN MEN DESIRE....

Being desirable is a quality women don't have to be born with—but one they can learn. Now erotic expert Graham Masterton reveals the secrets of how to talk, dress, and carry yourself in ways that will make you irrestible to men. And once you have begun a sexual relationship, here are the essential dos and don'ts of taking charge, setting the pace, maximizing the intensity, and giving your man—and yourself—the greatest sex of your lives.

Don't Miss Any of Graham Masterton's Other Sizzling Books of Erotic Instruction

All Available fr

D1059336

Secrets of the Sexually Irresistible Woman

GRAHAM MASTERTON

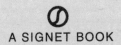

A SIGNET BOOK

SIGNET
Published by the Penguin Group
Penguin Putnam Inc., 375 Hudson Street,
New York, New York 10014, U.S.A.
Penguin Books Ltd, 27 Wrights Lane,
London W8 5TZ, England
Penguin Books Australia Ltd, Ringwood,
Victoria, Australia
Penguin Books Canada Ltd, 10 Alcorn Avenue,
Toronto, Ontario, Canada M4V 3B2
Penguin Books (N.Z.) Ltd, 182–190 Wairau Road,
Auckland 10, New Zealand

Penguin Books Ltd, Registered Offices:
Harmondsworth, Middlesex, England

First published by Signet, an imprint of Dutton Signet,
a member of Penguin Putnam Inc.

First Printing, March, 1998
10 9 8 7 6 5 4 3 2 1

CONTENTS

CHAPTER ONE

So You Want to Be the Woman Every Man Wants

What makes a woman sexually irresistible? Is it something she's born with—her face, her figure, the way she walks? Or is it something much more than that—an inner confidence that men simply can't resist? Is it possible, in fact, for a woman to *learn* to become sexually irresistible?

Tania wrote me from Scottsdale, Arizona, enclosing two photographs. One of herself: a pretty twenty-four-year-old with wavy blonde hair, blue eyes, and a very trim figure. And one of her school friends, Pauline, whom she had recently met at a class reunion.

Pauline was brunette, bespectacled, and slightly overweight (although by no means fat).

Two weeks after their reunion, Tania had taken Pauline to a party so that she could meet some of Tania's friends and business colleagues—including Jim, the accounts director. "I've had the hots for Jim ever since he joined the company," Tania confessed. "He is just *sooo* good-looking."

Tania thought that she was doing Pauline a favor by introducing her to some new people. "I'd gotten the

impression that she was kind of shy and didn't social-
ize much. And if you really want a true confession, I
didn't think that she was anything like as attractive
and outgoing as me."

However, Tania was in for a surprise. Her shy friend
almost immediately drew the attention of every man
in the room, including the sooo good-looking Jim. Before long, Pauline and Jim were enjoying an intimate
chat in the corner of the room while Tania was left talking to some of her girlfriends.

At the end of her letter, Tania almost howls, "*Why?* I
just don't understand it. I'm not trying to bring
Pauline down, but she simply isn't pretty. Okay, she's
quite big-breasted, but surely men are not attracted by
boobs alone. I have to say that I feel totally confused,
not to mention cheated. Jim talked to Pauline as if they
had known each other forever, and yet when I went up
to them he dismissed me with 'hello' and 'good-bye.'

"Later I found out that Jim and Pauline met each
other the next day and began an affair. I was crazy
with jealousy. I mean, what could Pauline possibly
have that I don't!"

You'd be surprised how often I'm asked this question (or something very similar) by girls who have lost
their boyfriends to other girls, by wives who have just
discovered that their husbands are having an affair,
and by women who consider themselves to be just as
pretty as every other woman they know and yet find it
almost impossible to attract the man of their dreams.

Without conducting a long and detailed psychological investigation, it's impossible to tell exactly why
one man finds you sexually desirable while another
one doesn't. Sexual desirability depends on so many
different factors, many of which you can never be expected to know. For instance, you may remind a man

of a former lover for whom he is still carrying a torch. Alternatively, you may have the bad luck to remind him of a woman who jilted him or who criticized his sexual prowess. You may remind him of a pinup that turned him on when he was fifteen years old . . . or a teacher who was always making him feel like an underachiever.

You may have some completely indefinable look about you that appeals to him. Your hair, your eyes, your voice, the way you smile—maybe they make him go all melty inside. Then again, there may be something indefinable about you that he simply doesn't like. Most of the time even *he* won't know why. These are all "X-factors" when it comes to trying to analyze why some women appear to be more desirable to men than others. Try to list the reasons why certain men appeal to you and other men don't, and you'll understand what I mean.

In Pauline's case, it might even have been her spectacles that attracted Jim. Contrary to what Dorothy Parker said about it—"Men seldom make passes at girls who wear glasses"—there are many men who absolutely go *wild* for girls in glasses. Peter—a thirty-five-year-old advertising executive from Baltimore, Maryland, told me, "My fantasy is making love on my office carpet to a tall, full-figured girl with long, shiny brunette hair who's wearing nothing at all but eyeglasses."

So . . . there are many "X-factors" involved in sexual attraction that you can never know and that you probably couldn't alter even if you *did* know. You can't change your height, your eyes, your ethnic origin, your taste in music, the way you laugh—and why should you? But there are many ways in which you *can* make yourself more attractive to the men you like . . . and, in fact, to almost *all* men.

I'm not talking about nose jobs or breast implants or collagen injections to make your lips look like Julia Roberts's pressed to a candy store window. I'm talking about ways in which you can talk, dress, and carry yourself that will guarantee that you will always stimulate sexual interest in men. I'm talking about walking into a room and turning every male head in the place.

I'm talking about being *irresistible*.

You can learn to develop your own sexuality so that instead of having to wait passively for a man to pay you some attention, you can draw him into a conversation, draw him into an encounter, and then draw him into a full sexual relationship, if that's what you're looking for.

And once you've started a sexual relationship, there are ways in which you can take charge of it, so that *you* set the pace at which it develops, and *you* control the frequency and the intensity of your lovemaking. From the moment you first make love, your partner won't be aware of exactly what it is you're doing to him . . . but he *will* be aware that he's having the greatest sex ever.

So many men are eager and passionate lovers—particularly at the beginning of a new sexual relationship—but so few men have a natural sense of sexual timing. They won't have an instinct for the right moment to kiss you, the right moment to touch you, the right moment to ask you to bed. You'd be amazed how many men try to approach an attractive woman and then give up because they've mistaken a little mild resistance for outright rejection—when, all the time, the woman was eager for them to continue. It's the sexually irresistible woman who has the knack of putting men at ease and encouraging their advances even when they lose their confidence and think they've blown it.

Men's timing is not much better even when you've gotten them into bed. Too many of them don't know how to stimulate you, and where, and for how long. And when it comes to intercourse (no matter how many sex education videos they've seen) they still seem to think that they're training to win the Kentucky Derby.

Good sexual timing can transform an average sexual relationship into a good sexual relationship, and make a good one brilliant. And the good news is that good sexual timing can be taught. First, you can teach it to yourself—how to arouse your partner more quickly, but how to make him stay harder longer. How to delay his climaxes so that you both have more fun. How to give him a second or even a third climax. How to make lovemaking last, literally, for hours on end.

With good timing and good technique, you can even give him a climax when he isn't erect.

Once you've learned good sexual timing, you can teach *him* good sexual timing, too—so that he knows when and where and how long you like to be kissed, when you like your feet massaged, when you like your breasts and nipples touched, when and how to stimulate your clitoris and your vagina.

Here's Helen, twenty-six, a grade school teacher from Philadelphia: "I had wonderful orgasms when I *did* have orgasms, but the problem used to be that it took me so long to get aroused. Most of the men in my life had finished and fallen asleep by the time I was only a quarter of the way there. Well, I say 'men,' but I only had three serious relationships from the time I was eighteen till the time I met my present significant other, Charles. I used to get so frustrated that I almost gave up sex altogether, and of course that meant that my relationships always used to come to a very argumentative end.

"With the first man I went with, I was too shy to discuss how I felt. I managed to tell the second man how I felt, but he thought I was criticizing his sexual technique, and *that* affair ended in a very nasty row, with china being thrown around the room. The third man simply didn't understand, unless he didn't *want* to understand. I struggled for a half hour to explain what I needed in bed, and all he did was shrug. I mean, literally, shrug. But right on the rebound from him, something terrific happened. I went to a party that was being thrown by one of my teaching friends and I had a little too much wine. At two o'clock in the morning I ended up in a motel room with Philip—he was a postgraduate philosophy student from the University of Illinois.

"The point was, he was as drunk as I was, and after we'd been making love for a while he lost his erection. I told him not to worry . . . maybe it was the Lord's way of telling us that we shouldn't be doing this in any case. But he said, 'Oh, no, you're not getting away *that* easily.' He turned me over on my back, opened up my legs, and started to lick me, all around my cunt.

"I tried to stop him, but he wouldn't. He reached up and cupped my breasts with his hands, and played with my nipples. But his tongue went on and on . . . probing into my cunt, licking me deep between the cheeks of my ass, but most of all flicking at my clitoris.

"It took just as long as usual for me to get aroused, but Philip didn't stop. He didn't have a hard-on, remember, and all he was trying to do was satisfy me in another way. Besides, it was turning *him* on, too. He was sucking my cunt lips right into his mouth, and drumming my clitoris against his palate, and that gave me a sensation like I'd never had before. I felt like opening myself as wide as I could so that he could lick me everywhere, and so that I could *see* it, too. I wanted to see what he was doing to me. I reached down and pulled my cunt lips wide apart, and there was the tip of his tongue flicking against my clitoris and then slithering downward, dipping into my pee hole, and then plunging into my cunt.

"I was so wet that there was a soaked area on the sheet underneath me. I had never been so wet before; it was all over my thighs and running between the cheeks of my ass. Philip's face was smothered in it, too. It was even sticking to his eyelashes.

"I could feel that my climax wasn't far away. Philip changed position so that he was kneeling beside me, and I could see that his cock was stiff again. The head of it was swollen like a big plum and there was clear juice dripping out of the end of it. I thought for one moment that he was going to stop licking me and try making love to me again, and I didn't want that. I needed him to go on licking, you don't know how much. I could feel this huge warm feeling rising up inside me and even my toes were beginning to curl.

"I reached out with one hand and slowly stroked his cock and his balls. He shivered a little but he didn't stop licking me. He had changed position so that he could slide his thumb into my cunt, and then work his index finger up my ass.

"None of my previous men friends had ever done that to me, and at first I tried to squeeze my anal muscles tight so that he couldn't get his finger in. But his finger was so slippery with juice that it slid right up inside me, and when he started to circle it around and around, the feeling was so strange and sexy that I didn't want him to stop anyway.

"He kept on licking and sucking at my clitoris, and then I knew that I was going to have a cosmic orgasm and nothing could stop me. I think I blacked out for a second. I didn't know where I was or what was happening to me, that was for sure. A great silent explosion of pure pleasure.

"I gave his cock two or three more rubs with my hand and he shot big warm blobs of sperm all over my breasts and my stomach. I lay back and slowly massaged my nipples with sperm and I felt like the cat who got the cream. Philip lay beside me and watched me and I'll always remember the smile on his face.

"I never saw Philip again. I found out later that he was married with two young kids and that apart from our one night stand, he had a reputation for being completely faithful to his wife. I have to say that I envied her.

"However—the most important thing was that I had discovered how to have an orgasm while I was making love. No more frustration, I thought. No more waiting till he was asleep and secretly masturbating. Three months later I met Charles, and Charles is such a terrific guy. He's funny and he's good-looking and he can recite practically the whole of *Hiawatha* without taking a breath . . . a pretty good qualification for somebody you want to go down on you every night, don't you think? But at first Charles was very—I don't know what the word is—*respectful*. He kissed me beautifully and he caressed my breasts beautifully. The second or third time we made love he actually went down on me and it was great . . . except that he stopped after a couple of minutes and climbed on top of me. I told him 'I love it when you do that, it really turns me on,' but he didn't do it the next time or the next and I didn't know what to do. I could hardly push my cunt into his face and say, 'Go on, lick me!' could I? Well, I suppose I *could* have, but even when you're having a sexual relationship with somebody it takes time to get to know how they're going to react, doesn't it? I might have put him off forever, and I didn't want that.

"I liked Charles a whole lot. In fact, I was falling in love with him. But every trip to bed ended up the same . . . with me feeling unsatisfied.

"It was then that I heard a couple of friends talking about one of your articles in *Woman's Own* . . . the one in which you recommend that women encourage their partners to give them more oral sex by shaving their pubic hair. One of my friends said that she'd tried it, and her husband wouldn't leave her alone! She said if only he kissed her on the mouth half as much as he kissed her cunt!

"I suddenly thought of trying the same thing with Charles. After all, my pubic hair was blonde, but it was quite bushy. It had never occurred to me to trim it before. Anyhow, I went home that evening and before Charles came over I took a shower. I snipped my pubic hair with nail scissors, and then I soaped my cunt all over and carefully shaved it, until I didn't have any hair at all. I looked at myself in the mirror and I was pleased with the way it looked—just two plump bare lips with my clitoris peeking out. It made me realize how neat and pretty your cunt actually looks; in fact, it quite turned me on, and before I knew it I was wet as well as bald! I lay back on the bed and masturbated, holding up my hand mirror so that I could watch what I was doing . . . flicking my clitoris and sliding my fingers in and out of my cunt. I thought that it was hard to imagine a sexier sight that that . . . a woman's own fingers with bright red painted fingernails playing with her own juicy cunt.

"When Charles came around that evening he was looking tired and harassed. He'd had a pretty bad day. I was planning on giving him dinner and a bottle of wine before we went to bed but I couldn't wait. I took his briefcase and then I took off his coat and then I said, 'Come here.' I was wearing my white silk blouse, the one he really likes because my nipples always show through it, and my short black spandex skirt. I kissed him and took hold of his hand and guided it up my skirt and in between my legs.

"He didn't say a word, but you should have seen his face. He fondled my cunt as if he had never felt anything like it before, gently squeezing my lips like he was squeezing a nectarine to see how ripe it was, and then slipping his middle finger into it, right up to the knuckle.

"He picked me up—he actually picked me up, the first time he'd ever done it—and carried me through to the bedroom. He laid me back on the bed and tugged up my skirt. He opened my thighs like somebody opening up a book. He said, 'That's the most beautiful sight I've ever seen in my life.' He kissed my cunt and then he started to lick it. It actually felt more exciting now that it was hairless, because I could feel all the wetness. I watched him for a while. He licked not only my cunt but all around it, and sucked it into his mouth.

"Then I had to lie back, because the feelings that he was giving me were so strong. When I masturbate, my climax comes all in a rush. But Charles kept on licking and licking at my clitoris, touching me much more gently than I would have done it, and I started to have this incredible tightening-up feeling . . . much richer and warmer and *darker* somehow than the feeling I usually get when I masturbate. He stretched my cunt wide with his fingers and kept on licking. Every now and then his tongue stopped licking my clitoris and plunged deep into my cunt, or flicked around my asshole. Then he smeared his whole face between my legs, so that his cheeks were covered in my juices. He couldn't get enough of it. You'd have thought that he wanted to eat it, you know, like a watermelon.

"The feeling inside me built up more and more. I lay back with my eyes shut, squeezing my breasts and tugging at my nipples, which I always do when I masturbate . . . except this time I could use both hands. All I could think of was this fantastic flick, flick, flicking at my clitoris. Charles sucked my cunt lips into his mouth but kept on licking at my clitoris and it was then that I felt this *wave* roll through me, this huge dark wave, and I didn't know where I was or even *who* I was. Charles said I was kicking and thrashing around. He said that I screamed out loud but I can't remember doing it.

"That was the first climax that I ever had with Charles, although Charles didn't know it. But he must have sensed my extra excitement because he got all excited, too. He knelt up between my legs and his cock was bigger and harder than I'd ever seen it before. I took hold of it and gently rubbed it, and then I gave it a long hard squeeze so that the end of it went all red, like a plum. Then I opened my legs up wide and guided it between my cunt lips. It looked amazing, disappearing into my vagina. Because I didn't have any hair you could see absolutely everything.

"Charles went right up inside me until I could feel his pubic hair up against my wet, bare skin, and his tight balls up against my bottom. He filled me up so much that he made me shiver. Then he started sliding himself in and out of me, very, very slow . . . not like his usual rhythm which was just a quick flurry until he came. And of course the reason he was fucking me so slowly was because he was already turned on . . . all that licking had excited him so much that he was right on the verge of a climax himself, and he was trying to hold it back.

"I reached around him and clutched the cheeks of his ass in my hands, digging my fingernails in, and pulling him into me deeper and deeper, in the same slow, beautiful rhythm. That gave him the message that I liked it slow, I liked it that way. I touched and tickled his asshole, too . . . and then I licked one of my fingers and slowly pushed it up into his ass, as far as I could manage. He sucked in his breath. I think it hurt him, but he liked it, too.

"That was when I realized that *I* was in charge of what was happening . . . or, at least, I was in charge of *how* it was happening. And the result was that *I* was enjoying myself more, and *he* was enjoying himself more. That realization made me feel even more excited, I don't know why. But the lovely slow way that Charles's cock was sliding in and out of me, the way that his hair tickled my bare shaved skin, it made me so sexy and so pleased with myself that I could have laughed. I reached around with my other hand and worked another finger into Charles's ass, so that I could stretch it open. I pulled it as wide as I could, and he said, 'Oh, God, baby, I can't hold it anymore.'

"He took his cock out of me just as the first big burst of sperm shot out of it, all over my naked cunt and halfway up my stomach. Then there was another burst and then another. I put my hand down between my legs and massaged my cunt with it, rubbing it into my lips. Charles held my hand and we massaged my cunt together, our fingers all covered in sperm and juice. I guess you could say that it was symbolic as much as sexy. I'd discovered how to get Charles to satisfy me, without making him feel that he hadn't been very good in bed before. And all it had taken was a razor and a little nerve!"

Helen's comment that she had discovered how to teach Charles to satisfy her *without making him feel that he hadn't been very good in bed before* was a very important point indeed. The sexually irresistible woman is the woman who makes her man feel more virile and more confident, no matter what his sexual shortcomings might be. If his lovemaking is too perfunctory, like Charles's, you'll only make the problem worse by complaining openly about it. You'll make him all the more self-conscious ... whereas fluid, relaxed lovemaking calls for a man to forget about technique and concentrate completely on giving you pleasure and satisfaction. If he suffers, for instance, from premature ejaculation—climaxing too soon—there are ways in which you can help him last longer, but criticizing his performance isn't one of them. Quite often, your disappointment will have the effect of increasing his anxiety and causing him to climax even more quickly.

This is not to say that you shouldn't talk about your sexual problems. There is no substitute for free, honest, and open discussion about your lovemaking. But sometimes, when the problem concerns your partner's lack of sexual expertise, it isn't easy to tell him what's wrong without seriously denting his self-esteem. No matter how discontented you feel, you should do your best to avoid belittling your lover's sexual performance. There are few remarks more damaging to a relationship than, "Not only that, you're no damn good in bed!" So when it comes to improving your sex life, think positive, rather than negative. Don't think criticism. Think *enhancement*.

Another point that we'll discuss in more detail later is the way in which both Philip and Charles enjoyed ejaculating onto Helen's body. In Charles's case, he actually took his penis out of her vagina so that he could climax all over her shaved vulva. This is because men are very responsive to visual stimuli, and while they derive great satisfaction from ejaculating deep within a woman's body, they find it intensely exciting if they can actually *see* their own ejaculation. A staple of almost all pornography is the "come shot," in which the male actor withdraws his penis at the moment of climax and sprays his semen over the woman's buttocks, breasts, or face.

Even when they have ejaculated inside you, men enjoy seeing visual evidence of their climax. Nathan, thirty-one, an aeroengineer from Seattle, Washington, said, "There is no sexier sight than seeing the woman you love lying on the bed with her legs apart, still flushed from making love, smiling, and come running out of her pussy." Irresistible? "For sure, I had to make love to her again, couldn't help myself." And Peter, thirty-eight, a security guard from Los Angeles, California, said, "The first time Beth and I had anal sex she turned over and went to sleep. I stayed awake to read for a while, and when I turned around she was lying there with her leg slightly lifted and I could see my come dripping out of her ass." Irresistible? "I didn't want to wake her, she has to get up real early in the morning, but I couldn't resist sliding my finger in and out of her ass a few times, while she was asleep."

Now, of course, male or female condoms are essential every time you make love to a man whose medical history is unknown to you. This means that many men are deprived of the erotic pleasure of seeing your vagina or your anus filled with their ejaculate. But—as we shall see—there are plenty of creative ways in which you can give your lover all the visual excitement he needs, even if you're making quite sure that there is no risky mingling of bodily fluids.

The "come shot" hardly ever features in pornographic videos made by women, and many women complain that they find it very irritating if their lover withdraws his penis just before his climax. "It breaks the closeness, right at the moment when you want that closeness the most," said Naomi, twenty-seven, a nurse from Baltimore, Maryland. "It makes you feel as if he's only interested in getting himself off, and that he's forgotten about you."

But there are ways in which you can make sure that you're an integral part of his climax, and that you get as much pleasure out of it as he does. Helen did it, when she masturbated with Charles's semen as a lubricant, and Charles was encouraged to join in.

A woman who understands just how to use a man's receptiveness to visual stimuli is a woman who can make herself sexually irresistible overnight.

But let's get back to the ways in which you can educate your lover to love you better. Because once you know how, you can teach him when you like your lovemaking to be gentle and romantic, and when you like it to be fierce and furious. You can teach him how to play out your most intimate fantasies, and all of those sexual games that secretly you've always wanted to try but never quite plucked up the courage to suggest. Sex toys? Bondage? Wet sex? Mistress and slave?

He won't *know* that he's being taught. He'll only be

aware that—with you—he's a better lover than he ever was before.

The sexually irresistible woman not only understands a man's problems but she also knows how to overcome them—without him ever being aware that she is pulling all the levers and twiddling all the knobs. The sexually irresistible woman is passionate and giving, but more than anything else, she's *patient*. She doesn't sulk if her partner can't get a hard-on after a long and tiring day's work. She doesn't turn her back, seething with resentment, if he climaxes too soon. She doesn't snap at him if he brings her right to the brink of orgasm and then stops touching her. She knows how to deal with all of these sexual glitches, and more—and how to turn them to her own advantage.

Above all, she is a realist. She knows that no matter how romantic it would be if a man were to sweep her off her feet, carry her up the staircase of Tara, and make love to her for six hours with an unfailingly bone-hard erection, most men have neither the panache, the skill, nor the physical stamina to do that to her, and she must (subtly) show them how.

The sexually irresistible woman makes her partner feel that he's strong and extraordinary. That's why she's irresistible. The man who makes love to a sexually irresistible woman is the man who can lie back after making love and feel like a million dollars and change—in spite of the fact that it was *she* who decided what they would do, and how, and for how long. And if you're thinking, "Hold up a minute, here. *He* may feel like a million dollars and change. What about *me*?" The answer is that *you* will be the immediate beneficiary of his newly acquired skills. The more virile you make him feel, the more confident he's going to be.

And when you increase a man's sexual confidence, he will want to make love to you more often and—when he does—he will gradually learn to take the initiative.

Being skillful in bed and knowledgeable about sex gives you the power not only to satisfy your lover but to make sure that *you* are always satisfied, too. It also gives you another power that is just as important: the power to keep your man to yourself, because he's far less likely to cheat on you if it means risking the greatest sex he's ever likely to have in his life.

I talked to over 120 divorced and separated men about the reasons they had been unfaithful to their partners. Of course, simple incompatibility was a major factor—"She's a vegan but I can't do without my baby back ribs," "We were high school sweethearts but we just grew up, and when we grew up we grew apart."

But one of the main reasons they looked elsewhere was because they believed that the women in their lives weren't sufficiently interested in sex. "I came home late, feeling as horny as an antelope, and all she did was turn her back on me." "I held my pecker in front of her face and asked her to suck it for me, but she said I was disgusting and refused." "I tried to kiss her but she said my breath smelled of drink, and then I tried to go down on her, but she said my chin was too stubbly . . . so, in the end, I turned over and said forget it." And the most common complaint of all: "She was frigid, that's the top and bottom of it . . . she just didn't like sex."

When I talked to their deserted partners, however, I discovered that more than sixty percent of them said they were not just interested in sex, but *very* interested, while a further large percentage said they were *extremely* interested. The problem was that they were no longer excited by the kind of sex their erstwhile husbands and lovers had been giving them, and they had seen no chance of their sex lives ever improving.

"He used to give me a peck on the cheek and then immediately he started fiddling with my pussy. He climbed on top of me, grunted a lot, and that was the end of it." "He never once, in the whole six years of our relationship, told me right in the middle of sex that he loved me, and that I turned him on. I might just as well have been one of those inflatable women for all he cared." "I knew he loved me. He brought me flowers and candy every week. He bought me all of this sexy lingerie. He was always telling people that he was proud of me. But he was so clumsy in bed. He flung me this way . . . then he flung me that way. He seemed to think that sex was some kind of wrestling match. He would just be hitting the spot . . . making me feel good . . . and then he would suddenly change position, throwing me onto my back or onto my side, and all of that good feeling would be gone. I felt like screaming at him, 'For Christ's sake, keep still!' But the irony was that he thought he was so damn good in bed. I heard him boasting to a friend of his that he knew two hundred different positions for sex, and I thought to myself, yes, and I've been in all of them, usually on the same night."

Obviously, many of their sex lives had been ruined by a disastrous lack of personal communication. I wondered how many relationships could have been saved if the man had been able to improve his sexual technique or the woman had felt able to show him how. I'm making no excuses for men when I saw that too many women are suffering a clumsy or inadequate sex life in silence . . . and saying nothing until it comes to the point of divorce or separation.

For most women, the main turnoffs in their relationships were: (1) intercourse too fast; (2) only rudimentary foreplay; (3) sex too rough; (4) no kissing; (5) same position and location every time; (6) no erotic pillow talk or sexual compliments; (7) no postcoital cuddling or kissing or expressions of pleasure and satisfaction; (8) no attempt to satisfy the woman manually or orally if she had failed to reach an orgasm; (9) complete unawareness and/or lack of interest in whether the woman had reached an orgasm or not; (10) no attempt to give the woman a second or third or successive orgasms—either through indifference or lack of knowledge that multiple orgasms were possible. You'll hardly believe this, but one man firmly told me that he wasn't prepared to give his wife multiple orgasms. His reason? "I can't have them, so why should she?"

Some of the women had resigned themselves to an unsatisfying and mediocre sex life and sought to fulfill themselves in other activities—business or rearing their children or charity work, or some kind of hobby—something in which they could win the admiration and attention that their partners didn't give them in bed. Others had become frustrated and bad-tempered, and their day-to-day married lives had been characterized by constant arguments. Still more had become deeply depressed and lost their sexual self-confidence. They avoided lovemaking whenever possible—the notorious "Not tonight, darling, I have a headache" syndrome, which is simply a code for saying, "I don't enjoy having sex with you anymore, because you don't show that you care about me, even if you do."

The result, of course, was that the men in their lives were much more susceptible to the advances of other women . . . and in many cases, had actively gone looking for a woman who wasn't resigned or angry or depressed. They had gone looking, in fact, for a sexually irresistible woman.

Why do some women attract men like magnets while others don't?

In the course of writing this book, I've talked and corresponded with dozens of women who have had spectacular success with men. This doesn't necessarily mean that they've had hundreds of lovers. In several cases, women have regarded "spectacular success with men" as meaning that while they have had only two or three sexual relationships since they first became sexually active, each of those relationships was both exciting and fulfilling. This is the whole point of learning how to be sexually irresistible: it allows you to choose what sort of sex life you want to lead, whether it's twice-nightly threesomes with well-hung young studs only half your age, or passionate once-a-month lovemaking with the man you want to stay with for the rest of your days.

Too many women find themselves in marriages or long-term sexual relationships in which their sexual needs are out of sync with those of their partner. Jeanne, for instance, a thirty-three-year-old grade school teacher from Cedar Rapids, Iowa, told me, "I've always been the romantic type, I guess. My idea of making love is hours of kissing and fondling and playing with each other. Apart from that, I *physically* need long and gentle foreplay before I'm anything like ready for intercourse.

"Jeff, on the other hand, likes his sex quick and rough. We'll be lying in bed reading or watching TV and he'll suddenly make a grab between my legs. The next thing I know I'll be kneeling facedown in the pillow, my nightgown over my head, while he shoves himself into me from behind. He only takes a few minutes to climax. Sometimes he's even quicker than that. Once in a while, I'd love it if he took his time and really turned me on. I know he loves me, but whenever we have sex he makes me feel like trash . . . like an extra in a porno flick."

Surely she must find this hurried sex very unsatisfying.

"You'd better believe it. If I didn't masturbate regularly, I think I'd have a nervous condition by now. But I bought a big vibrator that I keep hidden in one of the drawers under the bed, and when Jeff's gone to sleep I take it out and slide it up me, and I can lie there for *hours* sometimes, pretending that a man's making love to me."

Hadn't she tried to talk to Jeff about it?

"I've never had the courage. Cowardly, aren't I? But Jeff seems to have the idea that he's terrific in bed and he's always putting his arm around my shoulders and telling our friends what a great marriage we've got. He's always had an ego. I think he'd be absolutely shattered if I told him he was useless."

Jeff is typical of a great many men who regard sex as a regular means of "getting their rocks off" and never consider the needs and the feelings of their partners. I've talked to several men and explained to them that they were not doing everything they could to ensure that their wives or partners were sexually satisfied. In almost every case the men were amazed. "She never complained," they protested. But it was clear from their reactions that this was the first time they had ever considered the possibility that their wives or partners might have different sexual rhythms or different sexual preferences or that they might have romantic feelings that needed to be satisfied, too.

Part of the problem is that modern sex manuals and videos might have become bolder and franker and more explicit, but they seem to have forgotten that sex is not just recreation, it's a way in which two people can express their need for physical and emotional closeness. As twenty-two-year-old Donna, a dental assistant from Cleveland, Ohio, put it, "I like to take Marty's cock right into my mouth and just hold it there, sucking it gently, my eyes closed. I stroke his thighs and his stomach and his ass while I'm doing it, just butterfly fingers, you know, and play with his balls. I can stay like that for five or ten minutes at a time. And it's just like we melt into each other. I don't know whether I'm any good at cocksucking or not—that's not important. Sometimes we make love afterward; sometimes he can't hold himself any longer and he comes down my throat. But we never hurry. We're not out to prove anything to each other. We're just trying to get close."

Modern sex manuals and so-called instructional videos say a whole lot about positions and body parts and orgasms and getting pregnant (or not). They talk about fantasies and sexual variations—bondage and threesomes and wet sex. Openly (and rightly) they deal with the threat of AIDS. Yet it seems they've forgotten about emotions. Your partner may be able to spin a hula hoop on the end of his penis. You may be able to sign checks with a pen that's clenched in your vagina. But—fun as they are, exciting as they are—sexual athletics mean very little unless they are fired by the mutual desire to show your partners just how much you care for their pleasure and their satisfaction and their general well-being. Good sex—irresistible sex—is all about *giving*.

Even sadomasochistic sexual games are enhanced

by emotional involvement. Putting nipple clamps on a stranger means very little, even if that stranger happens to be your partner. But doing the same thing with somebody whose feelings and needs you really care for . . . that's what makes it really exciting. Maria, for instance, a twenty-seven-year-old art student from Los Altos, California, said, "I love being dominant, and whatever you say about it, men don't mind at all. In fact they love it. You couldn't say that my current boyfriend, Raymond, isn't a real man, but nothing turns him on so much as having me spank his bare behind with my hairbrush—yes, the bristly side. Then I hold his cock very tight, digging my fingernails in, and give his pubic hair a good stiff brushing!"

Maria is a good example of the sexually irresistible woman. She makes sure that she gives her man everything he wants . . . even some of those variations that he fantasizes about but has never plucked up the courage to suggest.

Here's Melissa, a twenty-nine-year-old dietitian from Sonoma, California. Melissa is beautiful, with honey-red hair, green eyes, and a spectacular figure. Yet in eighteen months of marriage her handsome husband, Chris, had never once given her an orgasm, and she was already beginning to feel that her sex life was unsatisfying and humdrum.

"He's a great guy. He's dark and he's good-looking and his body is just terrific. All my friends thought that he was the sexiest hunk they'd ever seen. If only they'd known! Whenever we made love, I always felt that he was simply working out. He used to kiss me some, but they were all little kisses, like peck-peck-peck all over my face and my shoulders and my breasts, the sort of kisses you give people at parties. Sometimes he would suck my nipples, which always turns me on, but he'd only do it for a few seconds and then go peck-peck-peck someplace else.

"He used to do this for a while and then he'd climb on top of me, open up my legs, and push his cock right up me . . . no more kissing, no more stroking. Then he'd slowly pump up and down like he was doing push-ups in the gym. In fact, I think that was where his brain was when he was having sex—back in the gym. I felt as if it didn't really matter to him whether I was there or not. He never spoke. He never said anything sexy. He just went up and down at the same speed until he climaxed. Then he got off, gave me another peck, and went back to reading his hotel management guide.

"As I say, he has a terrific body, and his cock is just fantastic. He could keep it up for twenty minutes before he came, and after twenty minutes I was usually getting pretty worked up, you know—in spite of the fact that Chris was so mechanical. But then he'd always climax, and stop, and I was always left right on the edge of having an orgasm, you know, like somebody trying to climb a mountain and never quite making it up to the top.

"Our marriage started to get very shaky. I always felt depressed and frustrated and I really believed that Chris wouldn't have minded *who* he had married, provided they didn't mind lying underneath him while he pumped up and down.

"I tried masturbating. In fact I became a fanatical masturbator, doing it three or four or five times a day, trying to get some satisfaction out of it. Sometimes I'd be standing in the kitchen and I'd lift up my skirt and put my hand into my panties and bring myself to orgasm in two or three minutes. Once I did it while I was on the phone with my sister. Other times I'd use two huge cucumbers . . . I'd smother them all over with baby oil and slide one up inside my pussy and the other up my ass. I'd lie on my back in front of the bedroom mirror and gently play with my clitoris until I came. I was always looking out for anything that I could use for masturbating—like once I even used this big bologna sausage. I was sitting on the couch wearing nothing but a black sweater, pushing this huge red sausage up my pussy, and the dog was watching me like I was crazy. I think I would have fucked the dog if I'd gotten any more frustrated.

"Then one evening we went to a party at the hotel, and Chris latched on to this really stunning blonde girl who was wearing this little white dress, and when I say *little* I mean she would have been arrested if it had been any smaller. She was bright and sparkly and she laughed at all of his corny old jokes. He was all over her like a rash. When we got home we had a row to end all rows. I said that he'd humiliated me in front of everybody, talking to that girl all the time, but he said 'At least she had some life in her—I don't suppose she'd just *lie* there, the way that you do.'

"Well, of course we ended up sleeping in separate beds that night. I was so angry you couldn't believe it. But what Chris had said about my lying there really stuck in my mind. That blonde in the little white dress had probably thought that Chris's jokes were as corny as I did . . . but she'd playacted. She'd flirted with him, and fluttered her eyelashes at him, and he'd absolutely loved it. You know, I hadn't seen our sex life from *his* point of view before. And what he had said to me was true. I *did* just lie there, expecting him to do all the work . . . all the kissing, all the caressing, all the foreplay, while I lay back and enjoyed it. I was turned on, but I never *showed* him that I was turned on. I loved him kissing me. I loved him licking and sucking my nipples. But he didn't know how much I loved it because I closed my eyes and lay still and didn't react.

"That's why he never bothered much with foreplay. And, of course, because he never bothered much with foreplay, I didn't get particularly turned on, and when he started making love to me it was just a chore for both of us.

"It's this really strange thing with sex, isn't it? You kind of assume that your partner knows how you're feeling, and when they don't it comes as a total surprise."

Melissa determined to change her sex life before it was too late. "That same night, I went to the spare bedroom where Chris was sleeping. I was naked except for a black garter belt and black stockings and black high-heel shoes. I slid under the sheet next to him and started to kiss him. It took him a while to wake up, but when he did he couldn't believe what was happening. I said, 'Sshh . . . don't say anything . . . this is a rape.' I sat astride his chest and kissed him long and deep. I didn't hurry . . . I wanted both of us to get totally turned on.

"Actually, I was turned on already. My cunt was wet and I was pressing it against the hairs on his chest so that they were wet, too. I reached around behind me and I took hold of Chris's cock. It was so long and hard that when I cupped his balls in my hand his cock reached halfway up my arm. I slowly massaged it and it seemed to grow even bigger. And this time I didn't forget to wriggle my hips and murmur and pant and I *know* that it was a little bit of playacting but at least it showed him that I was excited.

"I turned around and knelt astride him and took his cock in my mouth. It was so big that it almost choked me but it was all smothered in this delicious briny juice and I gave it a long hard suck and went 'Mmmmmmm,' so that he'd know how sexy and tasty it was.

"You wouldn't believe the difference in the way that he made love to me. He took hold of my garters and pulled me toward him so that he could lick me between my legs. I said 'ohhhhhh' when his tongue touched my clitoris, and wriggled my hips. As I say, I was only playacting—or at least it was only playacting to begin with. But after a while it turned me on, too. I was actually showing my feelings, letting them out, instead of bottling them all up inside of me.

"I sucked his cock as deep as I could. I dug my fingernails into the skin of his balls and tugged at them, and he winced and said ouch but he didn't stop me. All the time his tongue was lapping between my legs and it felt fantastic. I felt that I could do anything. It was like I didn't have any inhibitions at all. I took his cock out of my mouth and rolled it against my face, kissing it and biting it. I even gave it butterfly kisses with my eyelashes. Then I rubbed it against my breasts and squeezed it into my cleavage.

"I turned around again, and sat right over him. The room was quite dark but I could see him smiling at me and he was so damn *excited*, you know? I stretched open my pussy with my fingers and sat on top of his enormous cock, and this time I didn't have to do any playacting. It was so big, his cock, I didn't know how I was going to get it all in. But I slowly sat down on it, and it slid right up inside me, right up to the balls, and I let out this long, long sigh. Then I had to go eeek! because his cock had gone in so far that it had touched the neck of my womb and made me jump.

"We made love so slowly that it seemed to go on all night. We kissed each other and sucked each other and fucked each other. I must have had at least three orgasms, and a whole lot of little shuddery ones in between. Chris had his first climax when I was sitting on top of him, and then later I sucked him and slowly rubbed his cock until he had another one. It all dribbled down my fingers and I licked it off . . . and I didn't forget to make all the right *yum-yum* noises, because his sperm was delicious. Our whole love life had turned out delicious, as a matter of fact. We lay back arm in arm and we hadn't been so pleased or excited since we first met."

Melissa's experience was a prime example of how much you can improve your sex life by exaggerating your responses and making it crystal-clear to your partner how much he excites you. I know that sexual arousal is a very internal experience—particularly when you come close to orgasm. If you watch videos of women masturbating—such as Betty Dodson's *Self-loving*—you can see how your sexual personality closes in on itself as your excitement mounts. Your eyes close, your facial expression becomes more rigid, your muscles tense, your feet curl. But any way in which you can communicate to your partner the strength of your feelings will arouse and gratify him even more. Panting, gasping, screaming even. Or—if you prefer to be quiet—staring into his eyes with as much erotic intensity as you can muster.

At the beginning of this chapter, you remember how Tania was mystified by the sexual allure of her girlfriend Pauline? Without having seen Pauline in action, I think I can fairly guess that Pauline was the one who made eye contact with men, who listened to their stories and laughed at their jokes, and who, despite her apparent reticence, made it absolutely obvious to any man she liked that she was interested in him.

It's a knack. It's a trick. It's like Melissa moaning and gasping when she made love to Chris. But it's a technique, not a deception. All human beings respond well to being praised. How do you think an actor would feel if he gave the greatest performance of *Hamlet* ever seen, and nobody applauded? Next time he wouldn't bother. It's the same with lovemaking. The sexually irresistible woman applauds her lover with kisses and moans and squirms of delight. She makes him feel that he's giving her the best sex she ever had—and, in time, he probably will.

Now let's take a look at how you can walk into a room and turn every male head in the place. You're not scared to, are you?

CHAPTER TWO

How to Be Sexually Magnetic

"Where have all the wolves gone?" complains Georgina, a successful thirty-year-old doctor from Los Angeles. "These days, most men don't seem to notice that you're looking to get laid unless you take off all of your clothes and dance a fandango on the dining table."

Georgina, of course, is quite wrong. Men *do* still notice women, and they lust after them just as much as they always did. Some of them still come on hot and heavy, as plenty of women who work in offices will tell you. But on the whole they are a lot more cautious these days than they used to be. For a man to approach a woman with heavy-lidded eyes and a suggestive pick up line has become so sexually incorrect that very few men would dream of trying it anymore. Men have become much more reticent about approaching women for a whole variety of reasons, and the frustrating result is that while fewer women are bothered by unwanted advances, fewer women are bothered by *wanted* advances, too. Hence many potentially exciting and satisfying relationships never even get off the ground, and a truly staggering number of very attractive and sexy women end up without a lover . . . and without even an outside chance of getting married.

It's an incredible fact that fifty-four percent of American women between the ages of twenty-five and forty-four have never married and are not likely to, either. And an overwhelming majority of them report that their sex lives range from "nonexistent" to "spasmodic" to "fairly regular but not very satisfactory."

You have only to look at the columns and columns of lonely hearts advertisements in newspapers and magazines all over the country to realize how many women find it almost impossible to meet, attract, and then keep the sexual partner of their dreams.

One of the primary reasons many women have problems finding lovers is that their expectations are unreasonable. Ask a single woman what kind of partner she wants, and she will tell you that she is looking for a tender but strong personality. She is searching for sensitivity, confidence, and culture, all wrapped up in a financially solvent package of outstanding good looks. She wants a man who brings her orchids and takes her to the Four Seasons on their first date. She wants a man who takes her walking on the beach at sunset while violins play in the background and then makes wild and forceful love to her, murmuring into her ear the sweetest compliments she's ever heard. He gives her a multiple orgasm and leaves a diamond bracelet on the pillow.

Well, there's no harm in wishful thinking, but some of the best lovers are not the handsomest of men, and the types who look as if they might have stepped off the cover of a romantic saga are often the most self-centered and least considerate of companions.

What's more, the plain fact is that very few men are naturally good lovers. They are just as unsure of themselves as women are. Even today, with such an abundance of sexual discussion in men's and women's magazines, and regular programs on sexual behavior on daytime TV, they are still uncertain of what to do and how to do it. Quite apart from which, every woman's sexual needs and tastes are different, and when you start a new sexual relationship with a man, he's going to have to learn what it takes to excite you and what it takes to give you full satisfaction. Learning takes time. Maybe the last woman he slept with didn't care much for oral sex. Maybe she always insisted on sitting on top of him and bouncing up and down. Maybe she couldn't reach a climax unless she made love in total silence. You just don't know . . . and he won't know *your* preferences, either. Learning takes a little patience and understanding. So if your very first sexual experience with a man leaves you feeling frustrated, don't automatically decide that you're never going to go to bed with him again. You wouldn't stop seeing him if he took you out for a meal without realizing that you couldn't stand Tex-Mex, would you? So think about it for a while, and try to consider whether it might be worth showing him, or even *telling* him, what it's going to take to please you. Subtly, of course. You don't want him to think that he's inadequate in bed, and you yourself don't want to appear as if you're pushy and cheap. But no sexual relationship of any depth and real excitement ever came out of the fear of letting go. There has to be a moment when you take the plunge and risk a little commitment. The very worst that can happen to you is that you withdraw from the relationship—slightly battered, slightly bruised, but with the knowledge that you tried your best to light your respective fires.

The best that can happen, of course, is that you suddenly find that your love life has become the Fourth of July, every night. And that can and does happen— even between lovers who found at first that "our rhythms didn't match" or that "I didn't like the positions he wanted to make love in" or "he always wanted me to suck his cock before he went into me."

Sexually irresistible women are prepared to *work* at their relationships—right from their first encounter with a man they like. Much as you might fantasize about men being the hunters and you being the hunted, the era of cavemen and clubs has long since vanished. Women have become more self-possessed and assertive, both socially and economically, while men have become correspondingly less sure of their ground—particularly when it comes to a potentially sexual encounter.

To be blunt, they're afraid. Either of being rebuffed, and looking like a fool; or finding that you're getting too serious too soon, and that you're starting to discuss your wedding list after only one night in bed together; or of finding themselves accused of sexual harassment or date rape.

In the past decade the rules of sexual engagement have changed dramatically, and I applaud all of those changes that have given you greater equality and greater personal protection from unwanted harassment. But many changes have meant that you have to try just a bit harder to make it clear to the men you like that you're sexually interested in them, and that you're looking for them to respond. It has become more important than ever to be a successful flirt.

It takes skill, no doubt about it. You don't want to

appear like an old maid, and on the other hand you don't want to come on like a whore, either. But I hope the personal experiences that you read about in this book will give you that skill, and that by the time you've finished reading, you'll feel that you're ready to walk into any room and attract the man who attracts you the most. Or even attract a man you know already and with whom you've always been interested in having an intimate relationship.

Remember what I said about expecting too much. Many men conceal a great capacity for passion and romance beneath a reserved exterior. And often you will find that a man who didn't immediately turn you on with his jutting jaw and his athletic good looks will grow on you simply through the strength of his character and his sexuality. Nobody could say that either Joe DiMaggio or Arthur Miller was classically handsome, yet Marilyn Monroe fell for them and married them both. Nobody could say that Carlo Ponti was an Adonis, and yet he attracted and married Sophia Loren. One of my best friends has very little money and admits quite openly that he is "plug ugly," and yet I know from his beautiful wife that he is funny, loving, and very creative in bed. Sexual excitement has nothing to do with stereotypical handsomeness.

Maria, a twenty-eight-year-old receptionist from San Diego, California, told me that her husband, Juan, is half Mexican. "He's short, he's tubby, he has this droopy mustache, and he's very hairy all over. But ever since I met him at a party he's been the only man I've ever wanted to look at. He has such a personality. It's like a nuclear reactor. He makes everybody smile when he walks into a room. He's so giving, you know, and he's so humorous, too. He's always laughing. He's always making me feel good."

Maria admitted that Juan had another hidden attribute—"which keeps me very, very happy." Apart from his passionate nature, "He has the most enormous cock I've ever seen in my life—not that I've seen *all* that many. They say that size isn't important, don't they, and maybe it isn't, but I just adore Juan's cock. When it's soft, it practically hangs down to his knees, and when it's hard it's immense, with a huge fat head and a lovely curve to it, like a gigantic banana. If I suck it for him it gets really hard. I have to stretch my mouth wide open and I can hardly get my hand around it. He shoves it in so far that he almost chokes me . . . but what a way to go! And he seems to stay hard for hours. He loves to fuck me in the mouth almost every night, and then to fuck my pussy, and I love it when he fucks me up the ass for afters. That was so difficult to begin with, because he's so big. I mean it really used to hurt. But, oh, what a feeling it gives me now!

"All the time he tells me how beautiful I am and how much I excite him, and I tell him just how much he turns me on, too. I love it.

"Believe me . . . if I'd had to choose a sexual partner from a photograph I never would have chosen Juan in a thousand years. But good looks sure aren't everything, and if you asked me to give some advice to a woman who wants to find herself a man, I'd say that she ought to learn the art of looking further than skin deep."

Every woman has her own ideas about what makes a man physically attractive and what makes him a turnoff. One woman I interviewed while I was preparing this book said that she couldn't resist any man who looked like Al Pacino ("those sad Italian eyes . . . they make my hair stand on end"). And another woman confessed that she had a weakness for big, blonde trucker types ("especially if they look about ten years younger than I am"). Turnoffs included men with curly hair (don't ask me why), men with glasses, and "pouchy-looking" men "like Richard Nixon."

There's no accounting for taste, is there, and I certainly wouldn't recommend that you go to bed with anybody "pouchy." But the sexually successful woman suspends her prejudices when she first meets a new man, because she knows, like Maria, that even if he doesn't instantly appeal to her, he may have a whole lot more to him than immediately meets the eye. He could even have a concealed weapon like Juan's! Sometimes the shyest, oddest-looking guy in the room will turn out to be a much more passionate and considerate lover than the guy with the blue eyes, the suntan, and the perfect teeth. That's not to say, of course, that you shouldn't make a play for the guy with the blue eyes, the suntan, and the perfect teeth. But if you instantly dismiss a man's potential as a lover because of his looks, you're unnecessarily narrowing down your sexual opportunities—and you might miss out on the sexual experience of your life.

Now, you're going to think that I'm being a little bit unfair here. On the one hand, I'm suggesting that you don't make a snap judgment about a man the very first time you see him—that you give him the chance to show what he's really made of. But on the other hand, I have to remind you that men are very spontaneous when it comes to sexual attraction—and that a man will make a decision about whether he finds you sexually irresistible within the first few seconds of setting eyes on you.

Men are extremely *visual* when it comes to sexual response. They can look at a picture of a huge pair of breasts and find it arousing—even when they can't see the face of the woman these breasts belong to. Sexually irresistible women know that first impressions count. That means that it's very important that you're always well-groomed and that you've got a "sexual look" about you that men find attractive.

There are several sexual Looks to which men are especially responsive. You can look desirable and communicate your desirability by the way you dress, the way you fix your hair, the whole sexual identity that you decide to adopt. I'm not talking about being blatant. You don't have to walk around in ultrashort skirts or dresses with plunging cleavages. You can be very, very sexy without being obvious. But you can choose to give yourself your own version of one of the six Looks that men find particularly arousing.

In the ten years during which I edited two of the world's biggest-selling magazines for men, I instigated a simple but very revealing study of men's tastes in women's sexual looks. We did this by counting the letters we received each month praising the looks of the girls who appeared in our pages. Remember that very few readers ever take the trouble to write to a magazine . . . advertising statistics show that for every one hundred readers who feel strongly about something they have read or seen, only one will actually write to say so. Even to receive four or five letters praising a particular girl was a strong indicator that our readers found her exceptionally attractive.

Obviously my main interest at the time was to see which types of women would increase our circulation figures. But later, when it came to dealing with the ins and outs of sexual relationships, I found the results remarkably useful when considering how women could attract sexual partners more effectively. I suggested to several women who were having difficulty finding a partner that if they adapted their appearance to give themselves one of the six most popular Looks, they might have greater success . . . and, mostly, they did.

When considering the Look that might work for the best for you, remember that it's important not to try to be somebody you're not. If you're thirty-five and a successful, strong career woman, it's no use trying to pretend that you're a waiflike sex kitten. If you're twenty-three and dithery, it's no use trying to appear as if you're a calm, controlled secretary type.

Be realistic about your age and your physical appearance. Women always look sexier when they are making the best of what they look like. Overweight? It doesn't matter, if you dress well and act confident. Small-breasted? Who cares—you'll be able to flaunt it. Too tall? Too short? There's no such thing. Whatever you like least about your body, think positive. It's part of you, and you're beautiful, and there is always a way of dressing and behaving and carrying yourself that will make the most of what you have and what you don't. How many times have you seen a woman with a large bosom going to ridiculous extremes to conceal it—which only draws attention to it all the more? By the same token, how many women have you seen with very large bottoms who mistakenly think that Lycra leggings have some magical property for reducing the apparent size of their buns?

Making yourself sexy is all to do with enhancing yourself, not hiding yourself. When you walk into that room and see that man that you fancy, you don't want to have half your mind on how fat you are, or how much you hate your nose. *He* won't be looking at the small bump on the bridge of your nose which—in your eyes—is the size of Mount Baldy. *He* won't be looking at your hips and wondering whether you have to walk through doors sideways. He'll be looking at a woman who smiles, a woman who makes eye contact, a woman who knows how to flirt. He'll be responding to a woman who shows that she's genuinely interested in what he is and what he does.

He'll also be looking at your Look.

The Waif: this Look is generally for the under-twenty-fives only, I'm afraid, although I've seen some twenty-seven and twenty-eight-year-old women carry it off remarkably well. The key to this Look is the long, beautifully conditioned hair—slightly raggedy and windblown if it's straight, brushed out fully if it's curly. The hair has to be accompanied by darkly made-up, dreamy eyes . . . but forget about anything else except the lightest of foundations. You're supposed to be looking pale and girlie, remember. You want to bring out his protective instincts.

The waif's lips are always sightly parted. She wears simple short cotton dresses or men's sweaters that are too big for her. She is always asking innocent questions that give men the opportunity to air their knowledge . . . but she doesn't pretend to be stupid. She needs help unscrewing pickle jars, opening wine bottles, and fastening her jewelry. There are few more effective flirtations than asking a man to tug up the zipper at the back of your dress or fasten your necklace for you. They both appear to be practical, harmless requests, and yet they involve physical touching and an unexpected degree of intimacy.

Waifs appear to be immensely impressed by the men they meet, as if they have at last found the lover/protector/father figure they have always been looking for. Their apparent innocence allows them to be quite "touchy" from the moment they meet . . .

holding hands, linking arms . . . and when they leave, they give soft, trembly kisses to the men who attract them, like dew-moistened rose petals landing on his cheek, instead of the brusque air kisses of usual social practice.

The waif always has an ace up her sleeve. She has something complicated at home that needs a man's expertise. A TV, a video recorder, an automobile that won't start. She makes a point of telling men all about it, and eight times out of ten they offer to come around and fix it. Six times out of ten, a simple repair job goes a whole lot further. . . .

The Free Spirit: this Look can be adopted by women of any age, and because of the floaty dresses and saris that it involves is particularly suitable for women who are concerned abut their weight. Younger women can wear their hair long, with bandannas or scarves or headbands. Makeup, again, should concentrate on the eyes, although a cheek blusher in an unusual color gives more definition to the face. Older women can braid their hair on top of their head or wear a scarf over shorter hair.

The free spirit wears soft gauzy dresses that are temptingly see-through—or she wears caftans or billowy blouses with decorated jeans. She always wears a lot of jingly silver and enamel bracelets. She is friendly and full of aura and very *calm*. She gives men the impression that she is at peace with herself, but that she is very giving and sharing. She has taught herself to read palms (which is another wonderful form of flirtation, involving hand-holding and touching and tickling, as well as giving a woman an opportunity to say all kinds of flattering things to a man she hardly knows).

The free spirit listens to men carefully and tells them

that—even though they might be involved in nothing more spiritual than tax accountancy—they obviously have great character and sensitivity. Her acquaintanceship with mysticism allows her to talk openly about Tantric sex and other erotic activities without seeming to be too suggestive.

Men are attracted to the free spirit because they feel that she is sensual but independent, and that she is unlikely to demand too much commitment from them. She has mystery, too . . . and there are few challenges that men find more provocative than the idea of unraveling a woman's mystique. To the men she finds attractive, the free spirit gives a small good luck gift when she leaves . . . beads, a flower, nothing more than that. She tells him that a gift always finds its way of returning to the giver, bringing its own reward.

If he doesn't take the hint that she is expecting to see him again, then he doesn't have enough intelligence to be *worth* seeing again.

The C&W Look: a great many men find the country-and-western look totally irresistible. You'll need bouncy bobbed hair and natural makeup to give you that fresh "Oh what a beautiful morning" appearance. Go for skintight denim jeans coupled with checkered shirts with the first three buttons undone and the collar turned up in authentic Doris Day style. And whatever you do, don't forget your big shiny belt buckle and your little high-heeled boots.

A Stetson isn't necessary, especially at social gatherings in the city, but they're fun, and it's surprising how many women look really good in them.

What appeals to men about the C&W woman is her apparent independence, strength, and personal freedom. Although men may say that they like to take charge of a woman, most of them are looking for guidance from *you*, and you'll be surprised how many men respond to the C&W look by asking you for emotional advice. What they won't realize is that your Look is cashing in on all of those movie images of Western women that they've lapped up since they were boys— and on all of those emotional country-and-western songs about heartbreak and tears and women with cornsilk hair.

A C&W woman doesn't have to restrict her conversation to horses and cookouts and the Grand Ole Opry. But she should try to give a man the feeling that she likes the outdoors, and that there's nothing more romantic than looking up on a summer's night and counting the stars. The C&W woman can be quite "touchy," too, because she looks as if she belongs to a culture in which women were naturally treated as equals. She should try taking hold of a man's hands and asking him if he's ever worked on a farm . . . because they remind her of her father's hands, broad and strong.

You'll notice how often I suggest that you try to make some kind of physical contact with the men you find attractive. It can be deliberate (like the palm reading and the necklace fixing) or it can be "accidental" . . . standing so close beside him that his arm brushes your breast. Even though the contact doesn't commit you in any way, you'll be surprised how often you win a positive response. If you touch a man it clearly shows that you like the look of him, not necessarily as a prospective sexual partner, but as a person with whom you have physical affinity. And touch can communicate so much so quickly. Imagine trying to explain to a man you've only just met that you find him very, *very* attractive, and you'll understand what I mean.

The C&W woman follows up her initial approach by telling her newly hooked man that she's having a barbecue for some of her friends next week and that he's welcome to drop by and taste her cooking. If he says he can't, she smiles and shrugs and says too bad. If he says he can and doesn't show, she enjoys the barbecue all the same. If he says he can and he does, then she has an opportunity to show him that she cooks good as well as looks good.

The Secretarial Look: when I was selecting pictures for *Penthouse* magazine, I found this Look was always remarkably popular. Even more than women, men seem to have that old romance-comic notion stuck in their heads—that every woman with a French twist and glasses and a severe office suit is, underneath, a seething volcano of suppressed lust. "Why, Ms. Marchant, without your glasses you're—you're beautiful!"

This Look appeals to men who like a challenge, and like to believe that they have unparalleled powers of seduction. The idea of taking off your glasses and letting your hair down gives them a sense of sexual power, especially if they think that you're wearing a black garter belt and black stockings underneath your sensible skirt. The secretarial girl turns the normal rules of seduction upside down by looking as if she could be stunning if only the right man were to come along and show her how.

The pictures we used in *Penthouse* were so popular because we made this particular sexual fantasy come true . . . except that they were only pictures, after all.

Of course there's a trick to the secretarial look. It doesn't work if you simply put on any old pair of glasses and pin up your hair and walk around in your frumpiest suit. If you genuinely need glasses, make

sure that they really do something for your looks. Try
out new frames—especially larger, lighter frames. It's
extraordinary how a good pair of glasses can flatter
your features—emphasizing your cheekbones or light-
ening a heavy jaw. You may never have thought that
you would read a book in which it was suggested that
changing your glasses can change your sex life, but it's
true. Cherry, a twenty-seven-year-old realtor from Lin-
coln, Nebraska, always used to wear the same type of
eyeglasses with heavy frames—almost the same as the
eyeglasses that her mother had first bought for her
when she was sixteen. She couldn't wear contact
lenses because of an allergy, but she wrote me in des-
peration because she felt that she was never going to
have a fulfilling sex life. "Whenever I go out with my
friends, I'm the ugly one who never gets picked up by
a man. I was a virgin until I was twenty-two, and after
that I went for three years without having sex with
anyone at all. I met a really great guy called Alan and
we had a relationship that lasted for three months and
I was sure that he was going to marry me. But then we
went to a party together and he spent all evening talking to another girl who was much prettier than me."

Cherry sent me a photograph of herself, and I asked
an eyeglass designer to superimpose a new pair of
glasses onto it—lighter and larger to emphasize her
eyes. I also asked a leading hairdresser to change her
hairstyle, because she obviously used her hair to hide
her face, giving her even more of a dejected, mousy
look. The result was astonishing. It was a case of,
"Why, Ms. Marchant—*with* your glasses, you're beautiful."

Cherry bought herself a similar pair of frames and
changed her hair, and within three weeks she had a
new man friend. "I don't know whether it's going to

be a permanent relationship, but I don't care anymore. We have the most wonderful sex, and I know now that I *can* attract men!"

The secretarial look calls for more makeup than the other looks, and a more startling lipstick. Shades of scarlet look good with neutral-colored business-type suits. However, make sure the suit itself is immaculate and *understated:* the more naturally cut, the better. I have yet to meet a single man who likes those shoulder pads that stretch all the way to California. Your nails should be immaculate, your jewelry discreet. You're trying to look *demure* here, with hidden depths.

The secretarial woman is a good listener, and she laughs at a man's jokes, but she isn't slow to show him that there could be much more to her than meets the eye. She talks about the things *she* likes, and when she mentions something that particularly interests or excites her—like a scene from a recent movie or a painting or a place she visited on vacation—this is when she briefly takes off her glasses and gives him that sparkly eyed look, and then puts them back on again.

The secretarial woman has at her disposal one of the greatest flirtation techniques ever—the speck in the eye. She starts to blink and takes off her glasses. She takes out her handkerchief and deliberately prods the tip of it into her eye to make it smart. She tells the man that she has something in her eye and could he help her get it out. He has to stand right up close to her, gently probing the corner of her eye, while she holds on to his arm to steady herself. It's one of the most intimate things that you can ask a stranger to do—and, believe me, plenty of specks have led to sex.

The Exotic Look: I don't think I've ever seen it mentioned in any book on sexual attraction, but many men are very strongly aroused by the idea of dating a woman who's racially different. I speak from personal experience. My own wife is Polish, with very distinctive. Slavic features that I found instantly appealing the moment I met her, and still do, although it's very difficult to explain exactly *why*. Maybe I'm just into cheekbones.

Your own exotic look will depend on your facial features, your complexion, and possibly your ethnic origin. If you have any ethnic features or ethnic background, you can use them to your advantage to give yourself a distinctive Look of your own. It's a great pity that so many women try to suppress or disguise their individual beauty in order to look something like the actresses and models we see on TV and magazine covers.

I've met a great many young black women who have made themselves look absolutely stunning by wearing clothes and styling their hair in ways that women of no other race could possibly do. The same for some women of Oriental origin. But all too often I see the same regulation bouffant hairstyle, the same regulation makeup, the same regulation suits and skirts.

I'm not suggesting for a moment that you walk around in national costume, but you can emphasize your looks by playing them up. If you have blonde hair and Nordic looks, be brave enough to experiment with a short bob, some simple, well-cut dresses, and some plain silver jewelry. I know a young Hispanic woman who stopped lacquering her hair into a helmet and grew it out into masses of gorgeous black waves. She also started to wear much stronger colors and big, bright jewelry. It did wonders for her confidence, and wonders for her luck with men. "I was much more myself . . . I was much more relaxed . . . I was much more *fun*."

Carole, a twenty-three-year-old girl of Burmese origin worked in an advertising agency in Cleveland, Ohio. "My first six months in the job I tried to dress like all the other girls and I wore my hair in a twist. Hardly anybody noticed me—and when I say hardly anybody, I mean this copywriter that I really liked. Then one day my aunt came to visit and she said she was very proud of me. "Look at you," she said. "You look just like an American girl now." Well, I *am* American, but I'm not a white American, and I suddenly realized that I didn't like the way I was dressing because I wasn't being true to myself. Or to my looks, either. So the next weekend I bought a pair of flappy black silk pants and a white silk blouse with big flappy sleeves. I bought dozens of shiny bangles, too. I let my hair down and it's *very* long—I can sit on it. I sprayed on some patchouli perfume. On Monday I went to work and I turned heads from the moment I walked in the door. And you'll be happy to know that the copywriter I really liked is now my boyfriend. He always introduces me by saying, 'This is Carole . . . she's Burmese,' and I know how special I make him feel."

You don't have to be a full-blooded Cheyenne to take advantage of having a slightly Native American look about you. The point is to make the best of your own appearance, and to make yourself look interesting and attractive and different.

There are too many ethnic customs for me to make any particular suggestions about how you can go about establishing that first, all-important physical contact with a man you like. But you could try saying that you have Inuit blood, and that you always rub noses when you meet people. You think I'm joking? I know a girl who tried it at a dinner party in San Diego six years ago and she not only sparked a very exciting relationship with the man with whom she rubbed noses, but married him, too.

The Voluptuous Look: it's a strange paradox that although so many women are constantly dieting, the truth is that men like curvy, voluptuous women. You only have to look through the pages of any men's magazine to see that none of the models could exactly be described as sticklike, and many of them are positively enormous.

I'm not advocating that you abandon all control over your eating. It's not healthy to be overweight, and there's a difference between voluptuousness and plain old fatness. But if you have a fuller figure, don't try to hide it under oversized sweaters and tentlike tops. You'll only draw attention to the fact that you're lacking in confidence and that you have a low opinion of yourself. And if *you* have a low opinion of the way you look, how do you expect a man to feel about it? If a man likes you, he doesn't want to have to spend the first few hours of your relationship trying to reassure you that he finds you attractive and that, no, he's not lying to you and that, yes, he really does like a woman with big breasts and plenty of curves.

If you have a fuller figure, exploit it. You have only one life and only one body and if you're not going to be proud of yourself now, then *when*? Overweight is one of those problems that can cause constant misery and depression, and it's one of those problems that feeds on itself. The worse you feel about yourself, the more you need comforting and the more you eat, which is why you got miserable in the first place. More than any diet in the world, you need to break the cycle by understanding that you're just as sexy as the next woman, and that there are plenty of men out there who would love to take you to bed, just the way you are.

Wear clothes that show your confidence in yourself. Avoid the overweight woman's uniform of bright Hawaiian colors, elastic waistbands, and billowing tops. Dark, subdued colors will flatter you much more and give men the impression that you take yourself seriously. A low neckline under a tailored suit always looks good—provocative but businesslike, both at once. Avoid stretch pants or leggings at any price. Although they're comfortable, they show every single bulge and lump, and they're desperately unflattering, even on thin women. Buy blouses and tops and skirts that fit you, even if you wince at the sizes you have to buy. For the fuller-figured woman, the key to looking sexy is to look *smart*. There is nothing more off-putting than that "I know I'm fat so I've let myself go to seed" look.

Look more serious and act more serious. Many overweight women try to compensate for their appearance by laughing and joking and always trying to be "fun." They don't realize that many men who would otherwise find them attractive are put off by clowning. If you respect yourself and your own sexuality, men will, too. Remember: if you see a man that you really like, your weight is not an issue. Being yourself is all that matters. Being attractive is all that matters. Take particular care with your hair: a sympathetic hairstyle can make all the difference to the way you look. Emphasize your good points, paying particular attention to your eyes and your lips. If you have big breasts, flaunt them. Men love big breasts. If your waistline isn't as trim as you would like it to be, don't worry. Simply cut clothes in subdued colors won't make those inches magically melt away, but they will show that you know how to dress well and make the best of yourself.

When it comes to finding yourself a man, don't make your size a priority. Don't think, If I lose twenty pounds, I'll be able to attract the man of my dreams. Dress well, act normal, eat a regular balanced diet, and stay calm. You don't have to worry about being attractive tomorrow. You're attractive *now*.

Don't forget that physical contact, too. Make sure that you stand close to the man you like, so that his arm "inadvertently" brushes your breasts or touches your arm. Wear an interesting necklace in your cleavage and tell him that it's a magical charm from Bali. Even if he doesn't pick it up to look at it, it will certainly concentrate his attention on one of your most attractive assets.

I wrote an article for *Woman's Own* on sex and the fuller-figured woman, and I received dozens of letters from women who had always believed that their appearance was an obstacle to a more satisfying sex life. Jeanne, thirty-one, a receptionist from Chicago, Illinois, wrote, "Your article gave me such hope!! I'm not what you'd call fat, but I have a 44DD bust and I've always been very self-conscious about the way I look. I've always tried to hide myself at social occasions, but you're quite right. The more you try to hide yourself the more you stand out. So when I read your article I thought the least I could do was to try what you suggested. I bought myself a killer blouse and a black skirt and I had my hair fixed. The hair made all the difference, may I add. I always thought I had a big chin but the stylist brought my hair around my face so that it looked much softer.

"I was invited to a party at a neighbor's house and almost as soon as I arrived I was introduced to Paul.

Before my makeover, I never would have dreamed of looking at a man like him. He's very lean, forty-four years old, gray-haired, plays a lot of tennis, and is very good-looking. Usually I would have giggled and slapped him on the back and told all kinds of gags about being so busty. I used to think that men were looking at my body and nothing else. But I looked Paul in the eye and told him all about myself, and I listened to everything he said, and by the end of the evening I suddenly realized that because I had treated myself as being normal, he had, too.

"We had so much in common. We both liked art. We both liked jazz. I was actually *talking* to a man for the first time ever, instead of worrying what he thought about my size.

"I gave him my number, although I didn't expect him to call. But he did, two days later, and invited me to a jazz club. We had a great night and at the end of it he took me home. I asked him in for coffee, but we both knew that coffee wasn't what we had in mind.

"You read about evenings like this in romantic novels. He kissed me and told me that I was fantastic. He unzipped my dress and when he saw what I was wearing underneath he couldn't believe it. You always said to wear sexy underwear, didn't you? I was wearing a black basque and black stockings but no panties. And I'd shaved my pussy, too, just like you said. He couldn't even wait to take me into the bedroom. He couldn't even wait to take off my basque. He laid me down on the floor in the living room and he stripped all his clothes off. He has this incredible body, all suntanned and hard-muscled. His cock was standing up like a bone. I held it in my hand and rubbed it because I hadn't held a man's cock for so long. You'd never believe how good it feels, to hold a man's cock in your hand and know that it's hard because of you.

"Paul had a condom, thank God, because it hadn't occurred to me that he was actually going to want to make love to me. He tore open the wrapper and I rolled it on for him. I really loved doing that, rolling the rubber down his cock, and then fondling his balls as well.

"I opened up my pussy with my fingers, and Paul slid his cock inside of me. He kissed me and fucked me and it was heaven. I reached down between my legs and felt his cock sliding in and out of my pussy. He was so excited that it was only two or three minutes before he came. You can imagine that I was pretty disappointed. But he didn't stop there. He unfastened my basque, and took off my stockings, until I was naked. I have to tell you that I had never been naked in front of a man since I was twenty-five years old, and then he was always calling me names because I was fat. But Paul was all over me. He kissed my lips and my neck and my breasts. Then he sat astride me and drew off his condom, so that all of his sperm ran over my chest. He massaged it into my breasts and my nipples and I never felt anything like that before, a man's hands massaging sperm into your breasts and pulling at your nipples, too. I was close to having a climax myself.

"He kissed my stomach and my hips and my sides and my thighs . . . all those parts of me that I was ashamed of and thought were unattractive. Then he opened my thighs and kissed my pussy and licked my asshole, and no man had ever done that to me before. You can believe me that when his tongue went up my ass I was so embarrassed that I could feel my cheeks burning, but at the same time I was in heaven.

"Then his tongue went into my pussy and he licked

me, and all I could do was lie back with my hands clutching his hair and enjoy it. He licked me and licked me and I didn't even understand that I was having an orgasm until I felt as if somebody had suddenly hit me on the back of the head. After that I was shaking and shaking and Paul was clutching my breasts and I couldn't believe that such pleasure existed. I couldn't believe that two people could make each other feel so good.

"We did a whole lot of things that night, and most of the best things we did were *because* I was big, you know, instead of in spite of it. I remembered what you said and never apologized for myself. Paul loved my breasts and he fucked me in my cleavage and massaged his cock against my nipples. He loved the cheeks of my ass, too, and in the middle of the night I woke up and found that he was sliding his cock up and down between them.

"However good the sex was, the greatest moment was when Paul invited me to his company's anniversary celebrations, and introduced me to everybody as his new companion. He was proud of me, which I really appreciated. But it was you who showed me that pride begins with yourself."

I was flattered by Jeanne's letter, but most of all I was pleased by the way in which she was able to write about her sexual experiences. A few years ago, women found it extremely difficult to talk about their sexual needs so explicitly, but with the help of books and magazines and TV programs they are at last finding their voice—and their confidence, too.

Have no doubt about it—women with confidence win men and women with confidence keep men. Men are just as unsure as women about how to initiate a sexual relationship and they need encouragement and clear signals—just like the six Looks that we have just discussed.

While we're on the subject of attracting and keeping your man, I have to mention *The Rules*, by Sherrie Schneider and Ellen Fein. I don't normally find it necessary to criticize self-help books by other authors, because almost all of them contain valuable and constructive information. If you follow *The Rules*, however, you will almost certainly stay lonely and single for the rest of your life. *The Rules* advises you to always be demure and dumb in the presence of men, to avoid making eye contact, and to tell him nothing about yourself on your first date but your profession, university degree, favorite restaurant, and how many siblings you have.

You shouldn't accept an invitation for a date on the first request, and never for the same night. When he calls you, you should keep an egg timer by the phone so that you don't speak longer than three minutes. You should listen like an obedient Stepford wife to all of his problems—because he's paying to take you out. And you shouldn't sleep with him for at least three months.

Ms. Schneider and Ms. Fein completely ignore the fact that, these days, men are very quickly put off by women who don't show any interest. In the words of Chris Lafferty, a British computer programmer working in New York, "It's so demeaning. You don't want to appear a total sap." Peter Zorn, a New York banker working in London, said he preferred English women because they were more direct and more friendly. "American women are just into mind games. If women want to be equal they should enter into a relationship fifty-fifty."

The word "friendly" is just what I was looking for to close this chapter. If you choose a Look that's man-friendly, and you behave in a man-friendly way, you're almost sure to find a sexual partner of your choice. The authors of *The Rules* have made a fundamental error in confusing flirting with standoffishness. When you flirt, you can play hard to get. You can tempt and you can tease. But if you obey *The Rules*, men will simply think that you're frigid or incredibly old-fashioned or that you're playing them for an idiot. You're not supposed to sleep with him for three months? I slept with my wife the very first night we went out together and that was twenty-three years ago. I've met literally hundreds of couples who have said the same. They were immediately attracted to each other, and instead of playing girls' school games with egg timers they seized the moment. If you show a man how passionate you are, it doesn't cheapen you. If anything, you will earn his appreciation and respect. The sexually irresistible woman doesn't hide her urges under a bushel. She recognizes that she has needs and desires and she doesn't have to play by any rules except those of her own desire.

CHAPTER THREE

Please Your Lover . . . Please Yourself

When a woman is comfortable with her own sexuality, it really shows. She has a sexually attractive glow about her—but at the same time she sends out the message that if anything is going to happen, it's going to happen because she wants it to, not because she's been pressured or bullied or cajoled. She shows that she likes sex, but only on her own terms.

The critical difference between a *Rules* girl and a really irresistible woman is that a *Rules* girl relies on nothing more than the antediluvian art of prick teasing, which invariably makes men irritable and aggressive, while a really irresistible woman encourages the men she wants but *at her own speed.* The really irresistible woman is always offering something, but she's always clear what it is that she's offering, and how far she's prepared to go, and she isn't unfair to the men she's trying to attract. She never gives the impression that she's going to go to bed with a man if she isn't, but on the other hand she never gives the impression that she'll never go to bed with a man when, in fact, she wants to.

There is nothing that men dislike more than a

woman who plays around with their feelings, in the way that *The Rules* does. In spite of their apparent bravado, most men lack confidence with women, especially when it comes to initiating a sexual relationship, and the coyness and stonewalling that *The Rules* advocates belongs in some nineteenth-century drawing room, not in today's faster moving and much more honest world. There's nothing that men appreciate more than a woman being totally straight with them. Sexually irresistible women are straight, and that's one of the things that makes them sexually irresistible. Instead of refusing to take a man's calls, they'll come out and say, "I like you, John. I think you're funny and nice and sexy. But before I go to bed with you, I'd just like to know you a little better." What could be fairer than that? It leaves John feeling good. It keeps his libido simmering. And at the same time it gives you a while to make absolutely sure that you're doing the right thing.

One of the essentials of building your sexual confidence is to get to know your body and how it responds. As I've said, it's your body and it's time for you to learn to love it. Stop worrying about the things that you *don't* like about your body and start complimenting yourself on the things that you do. If you like, you can make a checklist of your good points: I'm happy with my breasts . . . my waist . . . and *very* happy with my legs. You'll be surprised that your good points far outnumber those things that you're less than happy about.

For over twenty-five years now I've been recommending self-discovery sessions, in which women can spend some quality time alone exploring their bodies and their sexual responses. Since then, many other therapists have recommended them, too, most notably

Betty Dodson, who has been called the Mother of Masturbation. In her self-love clinics, Dodson has taught thousands of men and women how to masturbate without guilt, and actually reaches orgasm along with her class.

She says that self-love is "the missing link in our understanding of human sexuality. Everybody pretends it doesn't exist, but the first form of sex we experience is with ourselves."

Self-loving is absolutely harmless and has many benefits. It helps you to know your body and how much pleasure you can get out of it, and because of that it helps you to like yourself more. If you like yourself more, you'll find it easier to be much more open and sexy with your partner. You won't mind dressing up for him in erotic underwear, or showing yourself off to him.

Vicky, a twenty-four-year-old receptionist from Denver, Colorado, said, "My parents were good to me but they were very conservative and sex wasn't a subject that was ever discussed in our household. I learned about sex mostly from the raunchy bits in Harold Robbins novels and what I picked up from other girls. When I was sixteen I had a best friend called Moira who invited me to stay over two or three times a month. We used to share her bed and talk about men all evening and what it was going to be like when we actually 'did it.' Moira said that one of the girls in our class had sucked a boy's cock. We both went 'yecch!' and I could hardly believe that a girl would really do something like that. But that night I lay awake for hours thinking about it and the idea of kissing and sucking a cock gave me a feeling like I'd never had before. I was still awake when I heard Moira making these little gasping noises. I could hear a sort of wet, sticky noise, and the bed was shaking. I turned on the light to see what the matter was, and there was Moira with her nightgown pulled right up. She was squeezing her breasts with one hand and her other hand was down between her legs. I knew what she was doing but I had never done it myself and I had never seen another girl doing it. I was shocked, I have to admit. But the incredible thing was that Moira wasn't fazed at all. She wasn't even embarrassed. She said, 'I was thinking about Wanda sucking that boy's cock. I just had to diddle myself.' I said that I'd been thinking about it, too. So Moira said, 'Why don't we diddle together?'

"I told her that I'd never done it before. I didn't know how. So she opened up her legs right in front of me, and said, 'Look, it's easy. I'll show you.' Well, I'd seen other girls naked before, of course, in the locker rooms at school, but a girl had never let me look at her like this. She pulled her cunt lips open with her fingers. Her cunt was very wet and red where she had been rubbing it. She put two fingers in her cunt hole and opened it wider so that I could see right inside her. I could feel myself blushing and I didn't think that I ought to look, but then she said, 'Look . . . this is the clitoris, here . . .' and she began to stroke her clitoris with the tip of her finger, going around and around. She said, 'If you lie back and think all kinds of sexy thoughts and keep on diddling yourself like this, you'll have the most wonderful feelings ever.' I lay back and I reached into my pajamas and started to do it but I was much too tense and I didn't really understand what I was supposed to be doing. So Moira said, 'Here . . . let me do it for you.' I said I didn't really want to, but she wouldn't take no for an answer. She pulled off my pajama bottoms and then she opened

my legs. She started stroking my clitoris in the same
way that she had been stroking her own. She said,
'Fondle your breasts . . . don't worry about what I'm
doing . . . fondle your breasts and think about sucking
a boy's cock. Just imagine it all big and hard and red,
and you're holding it in your hand. You're kissing the
end of it, and you're gently biting it, and then you're
opening your mouth up wide and sucking it, with
your tongue going around and around it.' She was
turning me on just by what she was saying, but her finger kept flicking at my clitoris and I began to have a
feeling between my legs like nothing I'd ever felt before. Moira slid a finger into my cunt hole, and then
another, and then another, and I could hear the same
juicy squelching sound that she had been making
while she was diddling.

" 'Imagine you've been sucking his cock and it's all
shiny and wet,' she said. 'He takes his cock and slides
it all the way down your body between your breasts.
Then he opens your legs and he takes his cock and
slides it all the way up inside your cunt, and it's so big
and hard that you can't believe how you've managed
to take it all inside you.'

"When she said that, she folded her thumb into the
palm of her hand, and slowly pushed her whole hand
into my cunt, right up to the wrist. Then while she was
flicking my clitoris, she wriggled her fingers inside of
me. I looked up at her because I didn't know what to
think and I didn't know what to say, but all she did
was smile. I guess that kind of reassured me that what
she was doing was all right. I mean it felt fantastic. It
felt like my whole insides were tingling. And it was
fantastic to see my cunt lips around her wrist and her
whole arm like disappearing right inside of me.

" 'Such a big cock,' she said, 'right up inside of you. You're all full of cock.'

"It was right then, when I wasn't even expecting it, that I had my first orgasm. It was like an earthquake, like shocks and shocks and more shocks. And all the time Moira was plunging her hand right into me. When I was finished she slowly drew it out, slowly and gently, and she reached down and kissed me right between the legs.

"After that, our relationship was kind of strange for a week or two. I began to wonder if Moira was a lesbian or something like that. But she kept on talking about boys all the time and it was obvious that she wasn't interested in making love to me . . . she'd just been showing me what to do. And I have to say that I did it. Almost every night before I went to sleep I would lie in bed and think about David, who was captain of athletics, and I would imagine what it would be like if I walked into the boys' locker room by accident, and there he would be, naked in the showers, playing with himself so that his cock was stiff. He'd come out of the showers, still wet. He had this terrific lean body, all muscles. I'd tug the towel away from his waist and kneel in front of him and take his cock in my mouth. That was my main fantasy right then. I was absolutely aching to know what it was like to have a big stiff cock in my mouth. I diddled myself night after night thinking about it, and some nights I did it two or three times until I was really sore.

"Then one day Moira asked me to stay over, because she had a surprise for me. I was kind of cautious about saying yes, after what had happened the last time, but Moira said, 'You don't feel guilty about it, do you, what we did together?' and I had to say no, because I didn't. She'd shown me how much pleasure I could get out of my own body . . . she'd shown me that sexual urges were normal and natural, and she'd also shown me that two women can masturbate together without being lesbians and without having any reason to feel guilty about it. Moira said, 'I like touching other girls' cunts. Cunts are beautiful.' And she told me all about some of the boys from the football team who used to go into the showers together and stand in a circle, masturbating. They'd touch cocks together, and rub each other's cocks, and in the end they'd shoot sperm all over each other's cocks and balls. They weren't gay. In fact they were totally the opposite. They just enjoyed their sexuality and had fun with it. Sometimes the boys even sucked each other's cocks . . . and you can imagine what I felt like when Moira told me that. A boy sucking another boy's cock, that turned me on so much!

"Anyhow, I went to Moira's house that Friday. We had a great meal with her parents and her kid brother and watched TV. But all the time I couldn't wait to see what the 'surprise' was. We had a shower and went to bed, and this time we were very daring and got between the sheets naked. We were hugging each other and giggling but we were both very excited, too. I'm not a lesbian, either, but I loved the feeling of our breasts pressing together, and I could feel that I was wet between my legs even before we'd done anything. Moira opened the drawer in her nightstand and took out a huge pink vibrator in the shape of a man's cock, with veins and everything. I almost screamed out loud! She said that she'd bought it mail order from one of her mother's magazines, and that she'd been offering to go down to the post office to pick up the mail every single day, in case her father collected it!

"We played with it awhile and wondered if men's cocks were really that big. But then Moira said, 'Close your eyes and pretend it's your wedding night. You're lying in bed with the man you love.' So that's what I did. I closed my eyes and tried to think that I was in bed with my new husband. It shows how innocent we were, doesn't it, that we assumed we would have to be married before we first had proper sex.

"Moira caressed my hair and then she started giving me little kisses on my lips. 'Darling,' she said, trying to put on this really deep voice. 'I love you so much. Your lips are like pillows. Your breasts are like pumpkins.' Of course that started us laughing so much that we nearly wet ourselves. But then Moira started again, and this time she played with my breasts and my nipples, and she stroked them with the end of the vibrator, and I could almost imagine that a man was touching his cock against my nipples.

"I opened up my legs and Moira started to play with my clitoris. I had such a strong feeling of anticipation, I wanted what was going to happen next, but I was afraid of it. It all seemed so forbidden and mysterious. But the feeling grew stronger and stronger, and then Moira slipped her finger into my cunt hole and said, 'You're so juicy . . . I think you're ready for me now.' She opened my legs a little wider and then she placed the head of the vibrator up against my cunt hole. I was dying for her to push it in, but she didn't, she waited for a while, and all the time she was playing with my clitoris and making me feel more and more excited.

"At last she slid the vibrator very slowly inside me, all the way up. She didn't switch it on or anything, she just used it like a dildo. She slid it in and out and all the time she didn't stop flicking my clitoris, light and fast. It was fantastic. I loved it. But I wished and wished that she were a man, and that the cock that was sliding in and out of me was a real cock.

"I had one of those climaxes that feels like it's going to snap you in half. I couldn't stop twitching and jerking. Moira pushed the vibrator even deeper up inside me and I didn't know whether I wanted it in or out. But in the end I lay back and when she tried to take it out I said, 'Don't . . . not just yet. It feels lovely.'

"After a while we changed over and I did the same to her. She lay back with her legs wide apart and her feet over my shoulders, stretching her cunt lips open with her fingers. She kept saying, 'Fuck me, fuck me. Come on, fuck me harder!' I was afraid of hurting her but that was the way she liked it. She wanted me to bite her and scratch her with my fingernails. I did give her a love bite on the neck, and one on her left breast, but I wasn't sure about the scratching. So while I fucked her with the vibrator, she dug her fingernails into her own bottom. She even pushed one finger up her ass. She must have been hurting herself because she made this hissing sound between her teeth. But it didn't take long before she had an orgasm, and she made such a noise that I thought she was going to wake everybody up . . . thrashing around the bed and going, 'Yes! Oh, yes! Oh, yes!'

"At the time I thought that what we were doing was playing childish sex games . . . but the surprising thing is that when I first went out with a boy that I really liked, and he wanted to make love to me, I felt quite confident about myself . . . about what it was going to feel like, and what it was going to take to make me feel excited. In a very gentle way, I was able to help him make love to me in the way that pleased me the most. And because I was pleased, he was pleased, too. I don't think I could have done that if I hadn't learned to masturbate, and if I hadn't played those sex games with Moira."

Of course, not very many girls are fortunate enough to have a best friend with whom they can not only discuss sex, but experiment with it, too. Vicky was a little worried about the lesbian connotations of her games with Moira, but at that age it is perfectly normal for one girl to have strong homosexual feelings for another (just as boys can), and even if she does discover that she prefers lovers of her own sex, her games will be just as beneficial in helping her to develop an exciting and satisfying sex life.

One of the valuable aspects of discovering sexual self-stimulation with another woman is that you can see for yourself how every woman is physically different and how every woman has distinctly different preferences when it comes to caressing, fingering, and penetration. Your genitalia are as individual as your face. Some women have very prominent clitorises, some have them almost completely hidden. Some women have large, convoluted vaginal lips, others have barely any lips at all. If you're interested in seeing how varied women's sexual organs can be, simply beg or borrow an adult video or a men's magazine, or watch Betty Dodson's video on self-loving, which graphically shows a roomful of women masturbating with fingers and vibrators.

There are all kinds of ways in which women prefer to be stimulated during sex. Some respond to strong, rhythmic clitoral rubbing; others like the fingers to flick lightly and quickly across their clitoris; still others don't like their clitoris to be directly touched at all. Some women like to be penetrated during stimulation—by fingers, or a dildo, or their lover's erect penis. Others find penetration distracting, and prefer to be penetrated *after* they have reached their orgasm—which often gives them the opportunity to have a second orgasm and even a third and a fourth.

Some women are very touchy about having their anuses fingered or penetrated, while others adore it. The most popular anal stimulation during intercourse appears to be a single finger penetrating the rectum as far as possible (a time-honored technique known in the eighteenth century as postilioning). But I have talked to several women who enjoy being anally penetrated by a vibrator during intercourse, and one thirty-two-year-old homemaker from Phoenix, Arizona, was a devotee of an enormous dildo that was two inches in diameter and almost eighteen inches long. "I can take it all," she said proudly. "If you can do that, then you'll know what it's like to be *really* fucked up the ass."

Now and again I come across groups of women who meet not only as friends and neighbors but to discuss sex and sexual problems and sometimes to masturbate together. What is noticeable about the women who attend these self-loving groups is not an obsessive interest in sex, but a calmness, a quiet self-confidence, a feeling that they're very happy with themselves. It's also noticeable that most of them seem to be contentedly married or living with a partner whom they love. Learning about sex and sharing your sexual feelings is a great liberator. So many women have nobody to turn to when they're worried that their partner doesn't seem satisfied with them, or that they're always faking orgasms, or that their partner might want to do things in the bedroom that frighten or alarm them. "He wants to tie me up . . . I mean, is that *normal*?" "He wants me to wear high-heeled shoes in bed . . . is that *normal*?" "He wants me to piss on him . . . I can't believe *that*'s normal."

Sometimes the unspoken problems are the worst . . . the feeling that your partner wants to do something different in bed but doesn't have the courage to ask you, in case you're upset or disgusted. There are many men who regard their wives as sacred and pure, and wouldn't ask them to do anything "dirty" no matter what. They would rather find another girl to satisfy their urges.

That's why it's good for women to get together and talk over their intimate problems, even if they don't go as far as masturbating together. It's empowering to know that you're not alone. It's empowering to know how other women feel—and how men feel, too. At a meeting of one group of seven women in St. Louis, Missouri, the members gathered on a king-size bed, all nude or partially dressed, and each in turn gave oral sex to the others, while those who were watching openly masturbated themselves or each other.

Davina, thirty-one, a paralegal and one of the stronger personalities in the group, said, "There isn't any greater intimacy that you can experience than arousing another woman with your tongue. It helps you to understand what it is about a woman's cunt that attracts a man so much. It helps you to know what it feels like and what it tastes like and the changes that it goes through while you get nearer and nearer to orgasm. It helps you to understand what *you* feel about it, and to be much more open about it. Some women still harbor a feeling of self-disgust about their cunts. They think they're wet and slimy and not very nice to look at. Once they've given oral sex to another woman, they change their minds altogether. They learn that what they have between their legs is a jewel, a treasure, and something that men prize above rubies."

One of the results of her oral sex sessions, said

Davina, was that all of the women encouraged their partners to indulge in it more often, and all of them reported an "immeasurable" improvement in their sex lives. "Women don't seem to know how to initiate oral sex," she said. "All they have to do is climb onto the bed and kneel either side of their partner's head, with their cunt within reach of his tongue. Do you really think he isn't going to get the message?"

My friend Xaviera Hollander ("The Happy Hooker") was one of the great practitioners of female-to-female oral sex. She once described a session she had with a girl called Nancy who came to ask her about a sex problem and then stayed the night. "I lay in her arms, feeling the warmth of her body and the rigidity of her distended nipples. After a few minutes of relaxing, I started to lick her, first her earlobes, then down her neck to her stiffened nipples, then all around her belly button, finally plunging into her delicious pussy as she gasped in pleasure. Her bush was heart-shaped, with the hairs cut fairly short. Holding each leg down with one arm, I started to flick at her clitoris with my tongue. She was soon ready to explode. Her arms banged against the headboard frantically, her head rolled from side to side, and low moans came out of her throat.

"I stopped and moved my head away for a moment, hoping to drive her just a little crazy. I could see that I was succeeding, as she grabbed my hair and tried to pull my head back down on her bush. I wanted her to beg me to start eating her again. I turned my body around so that my legs were near her head. Her thighs seemed divine as I spread them apart and once again began to eat around the small triangle until I hit the rose. I inserted my index finger deep into her moist cunt, then replaced the finger with my eager tongue.

"This time I moved my tongue very gently. She was so wet that I could really taste the juices from her slobbering cunt. I was so lost that I didn't realize that Nancy, in her own way, was trying to lick my clitoris and play with me with her fingers. She manipulated and vibrated my clitoris every imaginable way, then ended up squeezing it until it was almost painful.

"I turned around, facing her, and placed my leg between her thighs. Then I began a pumping motion, as a man would while fucking a woman, rubbing my cunt against hers. Soon I felt the first stirrings of what I knew would be a fantastic orgasm. I started to scream, and at the same time I could feel Nancy wildly pumping and having another orgasm."

Nancy had actually come to Xaviera because she was concerned that she might have lesbian tendencies. But after their night together, she went back to her husband, convinced that she wasn't gay. But her session in oral sex and masturbation had not only given her a clearer idea of her sexual orientation, it had strengthened her feelings of self-worth, and shown her, too, how she could educate her husband to give her the kind of multiorgasmic sex Xaviera had given her.

If you don't have a friend with whom you would feel comfortable indulging in mutual sexual exploration, then don't worry about it. You can discover your sexuality just as effectively on your own. Even if you're not married, or you don't have a current partner, self-loving will help you relax, and keep your mind and your body well-prepared for the time when you *do* find a man you want to sleep with. You may not be aware of it, but living without regular sexual release can adversely affect your temperament, increasing your stress levels and making you quick to lose your temper. People who have regular sex—even people who masturbate—tend to be far less prone to depression and to minor illnesses, and some recent research even suggests that they live longer, although other factors may well be involved (such as the likelihood that they're in a stable long-term relationship, with all the benefits of good eating and good domestic care).

In past books, I've suggested many ways in which you can get to know yourself sexually. Still one of the best is to set aside some private time for yourself to undress, shower, and pamper yourself with perfumes and oils while you get to know your body by examining yourself closely in a mirror. It's important when you do this that you know you're not going to be interrupted, and that you have all the time in the world. There is nothing more off-putting than thinking that you have to masturbate in a hurry before anybody comes home and finds you. It will only make you tense, which will diminish the pleasure of your orgasm or even inhibit you from having an orgasm at all . . . and what you're trying to do is feel comfortable with your body, comfortable with the idea of self-loving, and to give yourself the natural sexual glow that makes a woman irresistible.

Some therapists suggest that you make a date with yourself to masturbate . . . say six-thirty on Thursday afternoon, and that you prepare for it by buying sexually arousing videos or magazines, sexy underwear, and sex toys. In some ways I quite like the idea of that, because it helps you to build up a healthy sense of excitement and anticipation before you finally lock the doors, put on your favorite CD, and entertain yourself in front of your mirror. On the other hand, I'm a little concerned that the reality may not live up to the buildup, and that after your orgasm you may find yourself feeling disappointed and—yes—lonely.

Everybody experiences a sense of letdown after a sexual climax, and I would hate you to look at yourself in that mirror and feel empty and cheap.

Clara, a thirty-five-year-old fashion designer from Los Angeles, California, told me, "Every time I use my vibrator to masturbate I feel like throwing it away afterward. Like, what am I doing, pushing this horrible plastic thing up my pussy? Two or three times it's actually gone into the trash. But, you know, a few hours later I always retrieve it, and put it back in my nightstand. I guess most women who masturbate feel the same way. After you've had your orgasm, all your fantasies vanish, all those imaginary men who were fucking you in all kinds of incredible ways, they all disappear, and what are you left with? Just yourself and a disembodied dick. But that feeling doesn't last long. Once you've had a shower and a cup of coffee, you feel better—and you feel better than you did before you masturbated. I *like* to masturbate. I do it, what, two or three times a week—sometimes less, sometimes more. But I've learned not to be ashamed of it. I don't have a partner at the moment, and even though I know some great guys, I don't want to start a sexual relationship with any of them. So it's either no sex at all or masturbation. And, no, I'm not going to tell you what my vibrator's called. All right—Arnie."

If your time alone is limited by your job or your family schedule or the fact that you have children, then a one- or two-hour self-exploration session in front of the mirror is ideal. It's best to start by wearing at least a negligee or silky bathrobe. Sit down on cushions in front of your mirror and take a good look at yourself, at your hair, at your face. That person you see looking back at you is a loving, sensitive being who is interested in knowing herself and showing her love for other people. Remember what I said about looking at your good points, and not worrying about the things that you don't like about yourself.

Feel inside your robe. Feel your breasts. What kind of stimulation turns you on the most? Do you like gentle, circular caressing, with butterfly touches of your nipples? Or do you prefer deeper, stronger massage—and to have your nipples tugged and pinched? Do you think you could have an orgasm just from having your breasts fondled? Some women can. DeeDee, a twenty-four-year-old sales assistant from Council Bluffs, Iowa, wrote me to ask whether it was unusual that her boyfriend was occasionally able to give her orgasms after long sessions of kissing and playing with her breasts ("which he loves, because they're so big"); and Adana, a twenty-eight-year-old food store manager from Kissimmee, Florida, said that she was frequently able to reach orgasm by having her breasts rhythmically squeezed, especially if her husband waggled a finger inside her anus, too.

When you've aroused yourself by feeling your breasts, you can open your robe and move right in front of the mirror with your legs apart. It's important to have plenty of light, so that you can see right inside your vulva. You probably know what you look like already, but it's surprising how many women have never closely examined themselves "down there." Open your outer lips (the plump, padded lips with the hair on, unless you've shaved). There are your inner lips, coming to an archlike shape at the top, under which your clitoris nestles—that little pink projection that is the seat of your greatest sexual sensitivity. Touch it gently with your fingertip and see what it feels like if you try circling your finger around it, or stroking it rhythmically downward, or flicking it lightly as if you were playing pizzicato on a violin. Most women find that the sensitivity of their clitoris changes as they become more and more aroused. Some find that as they approach orgasm, they can tolerate quite strong rubbing, particularly since the clitoris tends to retract as climax approaches; others find that they need only the lightest of touches to bring them off. Your partner won't instinctively know what kind of stimulation you like the most, and when, so you'll have to show him. By stimulating yourself in a self-loving session, you can get to know just when you want him to touch your clitoris delicately, and when you want him to use the loud pedal. Remember—you don't necessarily have to *say*, "Don't do that," or "That's too hard." Sometimes a negative word can interrupt your lovemaking and spoil the mood. You can communicate how light or how hard you want him to stimulate your clitoris either by movements of your pelvis (moving it away if he's rubbing too vigorously, or moving it forward if his touch isn't giving you the stimulation you want).

Just below your clitoris is your urethra, the tiny hole that you pee from. Many women enjoy the sensation of their partner licking around their urethra, and very gently poking the tip of his tongue into it, but you should never insert any foreign object into it in order to masturbate. I once came across a case where a woman had inserted the tip of a Japanese chopstick into her urethra. She was lucky not to have suffered any internal injury or infection. It's amazing what you *can* do with your body, sexually, but at the same time you should always respect it.

Some women involuntarily release a small amount of urine when they climax, especially if their partner is on top of them and exerting pressure on their bladder.

However, others say that they derive extra pleasure and an extra sense of satisfaction if they deliberately urinate as they reach their climax during masturbation. Mostly it is just a physical release, but the pleasure also derives from having a climax that produces a visible result, like a man's, and from freely and openly doing something that, since childhood, has always been "dirty" and "forbidden."

Part of the enjoyment of sex is in the thrill of breaking taboos, as twenty-four-year-old Alana, a hotel receptionist from Orlando, Florida, discovered. "I wouldn't say that I was sexually repressed, but I was never very adventurous. I've only had three regular boyfriends since high school, and our relationships were very straight. No orgies, no bondage, no swapping partners, nothing like that. It was four months since Brad and I broke up and I guess I just felt a need to find myself—not just sexually, but in lots of other ways, too . . . like trying to understand who I was. I felt like I'd reached the age of twenty-six and forgotten to develop a personality.

"I was always good at English when I was in school, but I'd been growing up then and I was much more interested in boys. Anyhow, I made up my mind to start reading again, classics like *Little Women* and *Look Homeward Angel* and all kinds of stuff. Then I started a correspondence course in literature, which was great. It really made me feel focused. You don't realize how much books help you understand your own feelings. You suddenly realize that Jo felt exactly the same as you did. You're unique, right, but you're not alone.

"I started going to a gym class, getting fit, and I also started reading books and magazine articles about sex, because frankly I didn't know anything about it, and I wanted to know what I was like compared with other girls—or maybe if I was no good in bed and that was why all my relationships had broken up. I mean, unless you read a book or find another girl who's willing to tell you absolutely everything about her sex life, there's no way of telling, is there?

"Anyhow, I read your book and I learned about my body—you know, physically. One of the real interesting things you said was how to think about your vagina not as being a hole but as being an organ in itself, with a shape of its own and a whole way of reacting to being sexually excited—the same way a penis does, only it's much more complex and at the same time it's much more controllable. That really made me think of my femininity in a completely different way.

"I tried the sexual discovery session, too. It was a beautiful warm day and I had the apartment all to myself because my friend Sara had gone to Tallahassee to visit her parents. I went through all the things you suggested . . . pleasuring myself in front of the mirror, looking at my open pussy, touching myself, using a vibrator. It was then that I came across the chapter where you talked about wet sex, and women arousing themselves by pissing during lovemaking, or when they're masturbating. I'd never seen wet sex mentioned in any other book before. I guess I was vaguely aware that it was something that hookers did—'golden showers' or something—but that was all.

"I read about it and it was then that I realized that ordinary couples try it, too. I have to admit that the idea of it turned me on. I mean it *really* turned me on. Like when you're a woman you never openly piss, do you, not like men do. I was lying on this blanket on a big heap of cushions in front of this tall mirror which I'd propped up against one of the armchairs. I was completely naked. My poodle, Rex, was watching me and that kind of turned me on, too, being watched, especially since Rex couldn't tell anybody what I'd been doing!

"I started to masturbate myself toward orgasm, the way you suggest in your book. It took a little time, because I was self-conscious, I guess, and a little overexcited. But then I started to feel my orgasm building up, that fantastic tense feeling, and I started to rub my clitoris even faster and to massage my cunt lips, stretching them apart so that when I looked into the mirror I could see how wet my cunt was getting inside. I hesitated for a moment, because I wasn't sure that I ought to do it, but then I started to piss and masturbate at the same time. It was just incredible. I'd never actually watched myself piss before. It came out of my piss hole in a fountain that went right up into the air. It splashed all over the cushions and all over my thighs and my stomach and my breasts. There was even a puddle of it in my belly button. I carried on masturbating even more wildly and then I had an orgasm that almost made me black out. In fact I think I *did* black out, just for a second or two. When I opened my eyes I felt as if all the tension in the world had disappeared, and everything was perfect. I felt *free*, if you can understand what I mean. I was all wet and sticky but I was surprised that fresh piss doesn't smell bad at all . . . I even licked my fingers to taste it and it was just kind of tangy and herbal.

"I think it must have turned Rex on, too, because he came up and started sniffing at me, all curious and really aroused. He licked me between the legs a couple of times but then I stopped him. My cunt was quite sore from all that rubbing, and I think I'd had enough adventurous sex for one day!"

What was interesting and inspiring about Alana's

self-loving was that it was far more than sexual. At the age of twenty-four she had made a conscious decision that she was going to exploit her whole potential as a person—her mind as well as her body. She was intent on acquiring the knowledge that would give her both the inner confidence and the distinctive outward character that she felt she had so far failed to develop. Like so many other girls she had been distracted at school by the physical and emotional turmoil of simply growing up, so that when she graduated she had come nowhere near to exploiting her considerable personal abilities to the utmost.

I talk to literally hundreds of women who feel the same way—who have found themselves frustrated not just sexually but in all aspects of their lives. Like Alana, though, they have the power to change their lives for the better—by studying, by developing an interest in the world around them, by understanding that you never know all that you need to know, ever.

It's an old cliché, but with knowledge comes confidence, and with confidence comes the ability to control your own life, no matter what your present situation. With a wider knowledge of literature, Alana was able to form interesting opinions of her own, and to become a more informed and a much more interesting person for men to talk to. With a wider knowledge of sex, and of her own sexual responses, she began to acquire a magnetism that men found highly attractive.

"I had a sexual self-discovery session once or twice a month, when I gave myself two or three hours to masturbate and to try out anything and everything I felt like. I'd never tried anal stimulation before, so I spent one whole session dildoing myself up the ass, just to see what it was like. I taught myself to take something as big as a man's cock up my ass . . . so I knew that if it ever happened, I'd be ready for it, my body would know how to respond. I guess some women would think that what I was doing was shocking, or perverted, but it was exciting, and sexually it set me free. I don't have any guilt about it at all. If you can't do something really sexy and dirty when you're on your own, then when?"

At the risk of repeating myself, nothing that excites you sexually and that causes you no physical or emotional harm can possibly be construed as "dirty" or "wrong." I'm aware that some people consider wet sex repulsive, but many others find it liberating and exciting. Fresh urine is completely sterile and a moderate quantity can be drunk without any harm. In fact, some people drink their own urine for medicinal purposes.

Although anal sex is often regarded as "perverted," it is difficult to call any sexual act unnatural when it has been practiced in scores of different cultures for literally thousands of years, and when both men and women have a strong natural urge to try it and enjoy it.

We'll take a look at anal sex in more detail later, but for now you should be thinking about it during your self-loving sessions. Dr. Bernard Strauss, a urologist in West Orange, New Jersey, says: "There are many good reasons for healthy, monogamous heterosexual couples to experiment with anal intercourse. It can be a form of birth control, an option during menstruation, and, most important, the increased friction can increase pleasure."

For men, one irresistible aspect of anal sex is that it gives them the opportunity to boldly go where no man has gone before (even if a vibrator has beaten them to it), and men are still aroused by the idea of penetrating virgin territory. "He took her" and "He possessed her" are phrases that you often see in romantic fiction, but they have real meaning in male sexual psychology. For your partner to push his penis into your anus and think that he's the first person who has ever done it is a very intense turn-on.

So, of course, is the muscular tightness of your rectum, compared with your vagina. You can rhythmically contract your rectal muscles to bring him to orgasm without him even having to thrust in and out of you. And *you* will have a good chance of reaching a climax, too. Dr. Strauss says that "Women have orgasms comparable to vaginal orgasms," but in fact all orgasms are the result of the stimulation of the nerves in your genital area, of which the anus is part, so an anal orgasm is exactly the same, technically, as a vaginal orgasm—except that it has the added frisson of being the result of a "forbidden" act of love.

You can practice anal self-loving with nothing more than your own finger, lubricated with K-Y jelly or any cosmetic cream. If you don't own a dildo or a vibrator, you can try inserting a penis-sized carrot or a cucumber into your anus—although it's always safer to cover them with a condom, in case your tight rectal muscles accidentally break a piece off. I've had letters describing an extraordinary variety of objects that women have pushed into their anuses during self-loving sessions—candles, wooden spoon handles, rolling pins, flashlights, and rolled-up newspapers. A properly designed dildo or vibrator is obviously the safest and the most hygienic, and many mail-order sex-toy companies offer soft plastic "butt plugs"—with or without vibrator—that have a broad base to prevent you from accidentally losing them inside your rectum. You can also buy very thin anal penetrators, like flexible wands, that vibrate inside your bottom and give you the most extraordinary erotic sensations. For the woman who feels she can take it all, there is a slim penis-shaped vibrator, the "Slim Jim," almost eighteen inches long, that penetrates not only the rectum but the lower bowel. One woman described the sensation of dildoing herself with the "Slim Jim" as "being fucked up the ass by a very well endowed horse."

Your anus and your rectum are very sensitive and you should treat them with care. Always use plenty of lubricant and never try to insert anything into your anus that could hurt you or tear your sensitive internal tissues. When it comes to anal intercourse with a man, *insist* that he wear a condom, an especially strong one, too. The tightness of your rectum can lead to unexpected condom tears, as well as anal bleeding—and if your partner is HIV-positive, you run a very high risk of catching AIDS.

Understandably, many women are very reticent about anal sex. Some of them are worried because they think their partners are finding their vaginas too slack, especially after giving birth to several children, and are looking for a way to bring that virginal feeling back. Others are anxious because they think their partners might secretly be gay. Even more are concerned about cleanliness, or the fear that it might hurt.

A man who has an urge to have anal sex with you is certainly not gay. Almost all full-blooded men are aroused by the idea of penetrating your bottom, especially since part of the pleasure of anal sex is that they can play more freely with your clitoris and your vagina while they spear your anus. To those women who are worried about their vaginal size, they needn't be. With anal sex, there *is* the added bonus of extra tightness, but it can be very strenuous as well as exciting, and most men report that they regard anal intercourse as a variation, to add some occasional spice, rather than a main attraction. As far as cleanliness is concerned, the rectum usually contains no fecal matter, although it does harbor virulent colon bacteria. You shouldn't have vaginal intercourse directly after anal intercourse until you have taken off the condom and washed ... otherwise you could be exposing yourself to some rather nasty vaginal and bladder infections.

I spend a long time researching what it is that men want from women, and I have come across a rash of new sex phone lines that explicitly indulge the fantasy of anal sex immediately followed by oral sex. "I know it's filthy, but I want you to fuck me from behind, then let me lick your cock!" I have also seen several pornographic magazines in which women have submitted to anal intercourse and then lasciviously sucked their partner's penises.

There is never any harm in sexual fantasy, no matter how extreme it may be. But I cannot emphasize strongly enough that there are some sexual fantasies that should *remain* fantasies, and this is one of them. In all your sexual relationships you should be ultrafastidious about protecting yourself from AIDS and any other sexually transmitted infections.

In the first chapter of this book I talked about the importance of good sexual timing, and it is through self-loving and self-exploration that you will be able to discover what kind of stimulation it takes to bring you reasonably quickly to the point of orgasm. Of course, when you actually make love to a man the circumstances will be very different. There will be the added stimulation of his kissing and his touching and his affection. But it is important for your own pleasure and satisfaction that you know whether you need direct clitoral stimulation, and how much, and when, and whether there are other caresses that will help to arouse you, such as fondling your breasts or touching your perineal and anal area.

Some women find that they need very little more than the stimulation of a penis thrusting inside their vagina to become aroused to orgasm, while others always need additional fondling or rubbing of their clitoris before they are able to climax. The best way to discover what your needs are is to use a dildo or a penis-shaped vibrator during your sexual self-discovery sessions. If you're using a vibrator, don't be tempted to switch it on, because that will give you a false idea of how you respond to vaginal penetration. Unless they use a strap-on vibrator (of which there are various kinds available) the men you meet will never have buzzing penises.

If you are not one hundred percent certain about your prospective partner's sexual and medical history, you'll be using a condom, so unroll a condom over your vibrator to give you a similar surface sensation. Start by lightly lubricating the tip of the vibrator with a little K-Y or similar lubricant. If you're using a condom it will have its own chemical lubricant. If you're not, your partner will have exuded from the tip of his penis a few drops of clear, slippery fluid in order to facilitate entry into your vagina.

Don't stimulate your clitoris just yet. Relax, lie back, and slide the vibrator in and out of your vagina, gently at first, trying to stimulate as closely as possible the kind of thrusts your partner would make if he were inside you. Gradually build up the rhythm, and as you do so, watch yourself in the mirror—watch the way the vibrator slides in and out of your vaginal lips. This is what your partner sees when he makes love to you.

Try to imagine how excited he feels as he sees his penis burying itself in your vagina. Try to imagine how much you excite him and how much he wants to arouse you. Try to imagine his urgency as his climax approaches, his overwhelming physical and emotional need to ejaculate inside you.

As you become more aroused, you can close your eyes if you like, and let your fantasies become wilder. Here's thirty-one-year-old Gaye, a legal transcriptionist from Houston, Texas, describing the fantasy she always uses to increase her arousal during her self-loving sessions: "I like to imagine that I've met this megarich oil tycoon, and he invites me back to his mansion for the night. He has a huge baroque bedroom and a huge four-poster bed. He takes off my clothes but then he covers my eyes with a blindfold. He says it turns him on. He climbs on top of me and starts to make love to me. His cock is enormous . . . much bigger than a cock in real life. It fills me up so much that I can hardly take it, and his balls are enormous, too. They keep thumping against the cheeks of my bottom as he makes love to me. His cock goes up so far, I feel as if his sperm is going to come shooting out of my mouth.

"He changes position, and turns me over, too, so that he is fucking me from the side, and playing with my nipples at the same time. Somehow he feels different but I don't know why. His cock is still huge, and it slides up me so far that he makes me gasp.

"He changes position again, so that I have to kneel doggy fashion on the bed. He grips my thighs and rams himself into me harder and harder. I reach between my legs and I can feel his big hairy balls swinging against my clitoris. I dig my fingernails into them, and that makes him fuck me ever harder.

"Now he has me lying on my back with my legs wide apart and my feet in the air. He's fucking me really hard now, like a machine. In real life, I'm pushing my vibrator in and out so fast that it's almost a blur, but I have my eyes shut tight because I'm supposed to be blindfolded. He starts talking dirty to me, whispers at first, like 'You filthy bitch, you love it, don't you?' and 'How would you like to be fucked by five men, all in one evening?' and 'How would you like it if men could watch you fucking, and they'd be standing all around you, rubbing their cocks because they all wanted to fuck you, too?'

"Then he climaxes, and I can feel his sperm flooding into my cunt. I'm right on the edge of an orgasm myself, and I think I'm not going to get there, because his cock has started going soft. But then he snaps off my blindfold and I see that there are four other men standing around the bed, all naked, with their cocks in their hands, huge great purple-headed cocks, and they're all masturbating.

"The tycoon says, 'You didn't know this, but every time you changed position, you were fucked by a different man, and you'll never know who they were . . . five men, all in one evening.' The men stand closer and I reach up and touch all their cocks and their balls in turn. They feel fantastic, all hard and rubbery. Then one of them starts to climax, and his thick white sperm comes splashing out of his cock all over my breasts. Another one climaxes, too, onto my cheek, and his sperm slides down my neck. The next one shoots his sperm onto my stomach, and the last one climaxes right into my face. I smear the sperm all over my breasts and my body and lick it from my face. In my fantasy it always tastes like ice cream.

"Seeing all this has given the tycoon another erection (which is really me, sliding my vibrator into my cunt) and he takes his cock in his fist and pushes it into me. That's when I have an orgasm, with his great big cock inside me—so big that my cunt muscles can hardly even spasm."

Gaye learned from her self-loving that she was capable of reaching orgasm through vaginal stimulation alone, but it did take her anywhere from fifteen to twenty minutes and she needed to conjure up a strong sexual fantasy in order to help her climax. She also learned that if she inserted her vibrator into her vagina at certain particular angles, she was more aroused than if she simply inserted it straight. In particular, she found that if she used the vibrator to apply rhythmic pressure to the front walls of her vagina, she became so juicy that she sometimes thought that she had wet herself, and she invariably experienced a "huge, flowing orgasm."

What she was talking about was *internal* stimulation of her clitoris. The clitoris is not just a little bud on the surface; that bud is only the exposed tip of an organ that is normally about an inch long, although size and width vary from woman to woman. Rhythmical pressure on the inside of the vagina can stimulate the "buried" part of the clitoris and greatly enhance the secretion of vaginal juices and the strength of your orgasm. You feel the pleasure of an orgasm throughout your body. But the main muscle that contracts during orgasm is the pubococcygeus (PC) muscle. When you climax, this muscle goes into spasm—gripping your partner's penis (or gripping your vibrator)—and gives you the concentrated sensation of pleasure.

There was a time when it was argued that there was a difference between "clitoral" orgasms and "vaginal" orgasms—as if an orgasm brought about by anything less than full penetration was in some way less satisfactory. But exactly the same spasms occur in all of your orgasms, no matter how you induce them, although the intensity of your orgasms can be enhanced if you discover what arouses you the most, and if you show or tell your partner what kind of love play excites you the most.

It is remarkable how many women have never ventured to tell their partners that they wished they would stimulate them in a different way. Jennifer, forty-one, a beautician from Denver, Colorado, wrote me, "Your last book changed my sex life only in one very small way, but that small change has made all the difference to me and I am now a *very* satisfied woman. I never had the courage to tell my husband that he always rubbed my clitoris much too fast and much too hard. It meant that unless I was *very* aroused, I hardly ever had an orgasm, because his furious rubbing was distracting me so much. Sometimes he did it so hard that he made me sore. But I read in your book how I could change position and put my hand on top of his to slow him down and guide him without making him feel that he was making a fool of himself. And I gave all the right wriggles and murmurs of appreciation when he got it right. I had a blissful orgasm the first night I tried it and I've had blissful orgasms ever since."

It is also remarkable the number of women who don't even *know* what kind of stimulation will take them more quickly toward an orgasm. "I never masturbated when I was young," said Netta, a twenty-five-year-old homemaker from Cedar Rapids, Iowa. "My mother always brought me up to be a 'good girl' and to 'save myself for my wedding night.' I knew about masturbation, of course, because the other girls talked about it at school, but I could never imagine doing it myself. When Jim and I were married, I had never had an orgasm, and I guess I only had the vaguest idea of what an orgasm actually was. Then I was talking with one of my neighbors, Diane. She's a few years older than me and very outspoken. She was complaining that her husband was working on a major contract and that even though they still made love regularly he was always too tired to bring her off. She said she almost always had to masturbate after he had fallen asleep. I was shocked but I was curious, too, so I asked her what exactly it was that she did. She said, 'The same as you, I guess.' So then I managed to admit that I had never done it.

"Diane asked me more questions, and she must have realized then that I had never had a real orgasm. She said, 'If you don't think you'll be embarrassed, I'll show you.' She tugged off her jeans and stepped out of her panties. Then she lay back on the white leather couch in her living room and opened up her legs. I *was* embarrassed. I was *very* embarrassed. But at the same time I knew that Diane was showing me something real important . . . something I needed to know about.

"She beckoned me to come sit next to her, so that I could see everything. She had dark pubic hair, clipped really short in a little heart shape. She opened the lips of her vagina with her fingers and started to run the tip of her middle finger all the way up from her vagina to her clitoris in this really light upward stroking. She said, 'Every woman likes to do it a different way, but this is the way I like to do it, because it always keeps my clitoris wet.' Inside her vagina she was already juicy, and every time she stroked herself she dipped her finger into the juice and slid it up to her clitoris.

"Her vagina seemed to open even more. Her lips

started to grow very red and swollen, and her clitoris stuck out more prominently, too. She was so juicy now that the juice was running down between the cheeks of her bottom. She reached underneath herself with her other hand and started to touch her anus, sliding her finger in and out of it.

"As she got more excited, she closed her eyes and rubbed her clitoris faster and faster, but still very light—she was barely touching it. Her finger went deeper and deeper into her anus, right up to the knuckle, and stayed there.

"Toward the end she rubbed her clitoris so fast that her finger was a blur. Her face was clenched as if she was hurting, and there was a red flush between her breasts. She was wearing a T-shirt but it was so thin that I could see her nipples sticking up rigid. She lifted her hips, squeezed her thighs together, and then she shook and shuddered and said, 'Ah! Ah! Ahhh!' until she was almost screaming. Then after a short while she opened her eyes and looked up at me and said, 'What did you think? It's wonderful when you know how.'

"That was the first orgasm I ever experienced, and it wasn't even mine! But mine wasn't long in coming. Diane said, 'Your turn now.' I told her I couldn't, but she said it was just about the most natural thing in the world. She unbuttoned my dress and lifted it over my head. Then she took off my bra and pulled down my panties. I had never been naked in front of another woman before and I could feel myself blushing. But Diane led me over to the couch and laid me down. She said, 'You're beautiful; you always have to remember that.' She kissed me on the lips and then she kissed my breasts and my nipples. She said, 'Indulge yourself . . . find out who you are and what you want and allow yourself to enjoy it.' I didn't really know what she meant, not right away. But then I was too busy watching her as she ran her tongue all the way down my stomach.

"She opened up my legs and parted my lips with her fingers. It was a really strange sensation, thinking that another woman was looking at my vagina so closely. She took hold of my right hand and guided it down between my legs so that I could feel myself with my own fingertips. 'Now try touching yourself the same way that I did,' she said. I ran my finger up between my lips, but I was so rigid and unrelaxed that it didn't feel like anything.

" 'Relax,' she told me, but I couldn't. So she lowered her head and licked me between the legs. I didn't know what to do or what to say. I felt like getting right up and leaving, but at the same time there was something inside of me that badly wanted to stay. She licked me again, and then again, and that lovely wet caress was like nothing that I had ever felt before. Not even Jim had ever done that to me. 'How does that feel?' she said. 'That's upward, the same way I do it.' And she licked me again and again, dipping the tip of her tongue into my vagina and running my juice all the way up to my clitoris. She tried licking my clitoris downward instead of upward, which I didn't like so much. Then she tried licking it from side to side, and swirling it with a kind of circular motion. I was much more relaxed now. I was beginning to feel warm and excited and very, very wicked! Diane was giving me such a fantastic feeling that I didn't want her to stop. But she lifted her head and said, 'Now it's your turn . . . use your fingers.'

"I said, 'Please . . . don't stop.' But she smiled and said, 'If you want *this* kind of loving, you're going to have to ask Jim to do it for you. What you have to do now is learn what you can do for yourself.' I hesitated for a moment, so Diane took hold of my hand and placed it between my legs. 'Try to give yourself the same feeling that I gave you.'

"So I started to stroke my clitoris, so gently that I was barely touching it. I was tense and awkward at first, but Diane stroked my forehead and then she fondled my breasts, and I began to relax. It took a while, but in the end I managed to find just the right rhythm and just the right way of rubbing my clitoris, almost like strumming a mandolin, you know? I began to feel very turned-on indeed, a fantastic warm, tingling sensation. I opened my legs even wider so that I could touch my vagina with my other hand. It was all slippery and I slid two fingers into it to feel how wet it was. Diane ran her fingers up and down the insides of my thighs, and kept on murmuring to me how beautiful I was. She said, 'Imagine that you're on a stage, and there's a whole audience of men watching you . . . they can't keep their eyes off you . . . every single one of them has a hard cock, and some of them are so turned on that they've had to open their pants and take out their cocks and masturbate while they watch you. You open your legs wider and wider and some of them are so excited that they can't hold themselves back any longer and they start shooting out sperm all over their pants . . . you have them totally in your power . . .' I had never been so aroused in my life. I couldn't stop myself from gasping out loud and flinging my head from side to side. I was like my whole body was being tightened up in a giant vise.

"Diane slipped two fingers into my vagina, next to mine. I could actually feel her fingers inside me, wriggling against mine. You would have thought that my instinct was to rub my clitoris even faster, but it wasn't.

I slowed down, although I was pressing harder now. I couldn't think of anything else except the feeling between my legs and the fantasy that so many men were watching me. I was right on the very edge of having an orgasm. I didn't *know* that I was, because I'd never had one before. My thighs started to come closer together; I could feel myself kind of clenching up. And I still couldn't do it. I still couldn't get there. It was then that Diane opened my legs again, gently but firmly, and knelt between them so that I couldn't close them again. It gave me a really exposed feeling. I was naked and I was showing everything—not just to the men in my fantasy but to Diane, too. I rubbed myself harder and faster, using all five fingers, and it was then that Diane took her long red-enameled fingertip and slid it into my anus.

"I had an orgasm immediately. I was like a thunderclap. I was jumping and shaking and I didn't know what had hit me. Diane told me afterward that I was still having 'aftershocks' almost a minute later. I lay back on the couch and I was shiny all over with perspiration and panting like I'd run a marathon.

"Diane kissed me on the lips. She said, 'Now you know what it's all about; go home and try it on Jim.' I said, 'I have just one question.' She said, 'What is it?' I said, 'Where did all the men go?' "

Very few women are as lucky as Netta in having a friend as sexually liberated as Diane, who can show them firsthand how to pleasure themselves. These days, of course, there are countless instructional videos available that clearly show women masturbating in different ways. But there is nothing as valuable as the experience of actually touching and being touched.

I have found many groups of women who find it

both therapeutic and arousing to talk about their sex lives and to share their experiences and their fantasies. A few of them go so far as to explore each other intimately and to masturbate together. Joy, a thirty-four-year-old insurance salesperson, says she and three of her friends have regular "girls' nights" when they "eat pasta, drink wine, pig out on chocolate, take showers together, try on each other's makeup, talk about sex, drink more wine, watch sexy videos on the bedroom TV, and masturbate each other." Even oral sex like the St. Louis seven? "Sometimes. . . . Nothing tastes more delicious than a clean woman."

Isn't she concerned about her sexual orientation? "Of course not. All of us are heterosexual and all of us love men. But nights like that give us a feeling of being special . . . not just toys that were put on this earth for men to enjoy, but sexual beings in our own right."

So this is what self-loving is all about: not just learning how to excite yourself sexually, so that you can teach your partner how to excite you, too, but developing a sense of confidence in your own sexuality. Self-loving helps you overcome any fears you may have about sex and sexual variations, and is an invaluable aid to increasing your knowledge of sex and to discovering what kind of woman you are. It helps you to find out what your limits are, sexually, and just how much farther you might be prepared to go.

We'll talk about your personal sexual preferences a little later, but always remember this: you don't have to participate in unusual sexual variations to be sexually irresistible. I've talked to scores of women who find bondage a turnoff, who absolutely hate rubber and other fetishistic clothing, who don't particularly care for anal sex, who wouldn't urinate during lovemaking if you paid them, and who would run a mile if their partners came anywhere near them with a vibrator or a tickler or a string of Thai love beads.

Being sexually irresistible involves being sexually knowledgeable and sexually adventurous, but it certainly doesn't involve taking part in sexual acts that you really don't like, just for the sake of pleasuring your partner. If he's any kind of a lover, he'll take the hint when you tell him, "Please don't do that," or when you twist yourself out of his reach. It's important, though, that you don't make him feel that you're disgusted or that he's turned you off. After all, everybody has fantasies, and you can't really blame him for trying to make one of his fantasies come true. You just have to make sure that you immediately give him something in return for *not* letting him tie you up, or *not* penetrating you with that huge bright blue vibrator. Make sure that it's something that you really like, such as oral sex or squeezing his penis between your breasts, so that you can do it with obvious enthusiasm. He may be disappointed that you didn't want to do that very dirty thing he had in mind, but believe me, it won't be for long.

CHAPTER FOUR

What Women Secretly Crave . . . And How They Can Get It

Sexual self-discovery sessions worked wonders for women who previously had no clear idea about what actually happened when they became aroused. Also, they learned how they could educate their partners to give them the satisfaction they deserved.

"I had never really understood what I was like 'down there,' " wrote Kathy, from St. Paul, Minnesota. "Now you've made me appreciate how beautiful I am and what beautiful feelings I can experience. I am not a supporter of pornography in any way, but now I can appreciate how girls can appear in magazines proudly showing 'everything they've got.' A woman's body is certainly something to be proud of."

Many women find that sexual self-discovery sessions help them to develop a much more relaxed attitude toward lovemaking. "I was never one to experiment," wrote Lenore, forty-six, from Battle Creek, Michigan. "If you had ever told me that I would be dressing up for my husband in stockings and garter belt and wearing high-heeled shoes in bed, I wouldn't have believed you. But now I feel I can do almost anything and enjoy it to the fullest. It's like all of my embarrassment has gone.

Two nights ago, when my husband was on top of me, making love, I took my vibrator and slowly screwed it into his ass, right up to the hilt. I was amazed that he could take it, but it turned him on so much that his cock went as stiff as a broomstick. I switched the vibrator on and he came at once. To think that I wouldn't even have thought of *mentioning* something like that before, let alone doing it!"

Another value of sexual self-discovery sessions is that they help to take the fear and the uncertainty out of sex. "I was always kind of nervous about anything at all—well, *different*," said Eloise, twenty-six, from New York. "I thought I had a good sex life with my husband, Ted, but all our lovemaking was very straightforward. You know, him on top and me underneath. Ted tried to suggest other things but I wouldn't. Once he even brought home a sex video but I wouldn't watch it. I don't really know why, but if I saw a sex video or a magazine it made me feel threatened. I didn't think they were disgusting so much as frightening. It was like going into a roomful of people and they're all laughing and you can't understand what they're laughing at. I always felt as if I was on the outside looking in.

"I saw an advertisement in a woman's magazine for a sex aid called 'The Tongue,' which was a vibrator with an artificial tongue on the end of it. Afterward I couldn't stop thinking about it. I kept thinking, do women actually *use* that thing? I mean, do they really put it between their legs and let it lick them? I guessed they must . . . otherwise the manufacturers wouldn't have made them, would they, and they wouldn't be advertising them for sale. And this was in a perfectly respectable magazine.

"I mentioned it to one of my best friends, and she

didn't seem to be shocked about it at all. In fact she openly said that she wouldn't mind trying it. She actually admitted that she had a vibrator already, which she'd bought to try out during one of your self-discovery sessions. She said that she didn't use it much anymore: after her self-discovery session her boyfriend had said that she was 'one hundred percent hotter' in bed, and they were making out almost every night. She lent me a copy of your book and I read all about it, but I was still too uptight about it to try it for real.

"Weeks went by and I still did nothing, but then Ted and I had a real bad argument and we both said some things that we shouldn't. I said he didn't appreciate me and he said that when it came to making love I just lay there like I was dead. I can't tell you how much that hurt me. And it hurt all the more because I knew that it was partly true. I lay there and let Ted do all the work because I simply didn't know what to do, and I was frightened of doing something wrong and making myself look like a fool. Like I knew about oral sex, but supposing I tried to do it and it didn't turn him on? Supposing I couldn't get him to climax? And if he did climax, what was I supposed to do? Was I supposed to swallow his sperm or what? And what if it made me gag?

"After our argument, though, I made up my mind that I had to do something to change the way I was. I read about your sexual self-discovery sessions and I made a date with myself to try one. I chose an evening when Ted had to go to a conference in Pittsburgh, so I knew that I wasn't going to be disturbed. I clipped the coupon out of the magazine and ordered The Tongue. It was nearly forty dollars so I hoped it was going to be worth it! We still had the sex video and magazines that

Ted had brought home, stashed at the back of the closet, so I wouldn't have to worry about buying any of those. I bought myself a bottle of Chanel body lotion and a big box of my favorite candies and I was determined that I was going to enjoy myself.

"At last The Tongue arrived in a plain box and at first I was too nervous to even open it. But now I had everything I needed for a self-discovery session and I knew that I had to do it. I set up the living room so that it was all warm and comfortable. I spread a comforter on the floor, with a big heap of cushions on top of it. I took down the mirror from over the fireplace and propped it up against the wall so that I would be able to watch myself. I put on my *Orinoco Flow* album to soothe my nerves. Then I opened up The Tongue. It was much softer than I thought it was going to be . . . and when you switch it on, it has a kind of round-and-round motion. All the same, I was still feeling very anxious about using it.

"I took off all of my clothes and sat on the cushions in front of the mirror. I poured a little body lotion on my hands and smoothed it into my arms and my neck. Then I started to massage my breasts with it, watching myself in the mirror all the time. I squeezed my breasts until they bulged through my fingers, and I stroked and fondled and tugged at my nipples. I had never played with my breasts so much before, and I was surprised how arousing it could feel. In fact I didn't want to stop. I think I could have reached a climax just by massaging my breasts and gently pinching and pulling my nipples.

"I smoothed the body lotion all the way down my stomach and along my thighs. I was beginning to feel much more relaxed about what I was doing. I looked at myself in the mirror and I thought to myself, you're a very sexy woman, do you know that? I heaped up my hair with my hand and pouted my lips and I made myself laugh . . . but I *did* look very sexy.

"At last, when I really felt I was ready, I opened my legs. I had a lamp on the coffee table next to the mirror and the light shone directly onto my pussy. I gently parted the lips and looked at myself, the way you recommend. I could see my clitoris, my urethra, my vagina. I touched them with my fingertips, very lightly, to see what they felt like. Then I put two fingers into my vagina and opened it wide so that I could see inside. That was the first time I understood what you meant when you described a woman's vagina as having a shape of its own, just like a man's cock only *inside*, rather than outside.

"I opened up all of the sex magazines that Ted had brought home, and compared my pussy to the pussies of the girls in the pictures. You don't realize how different they all are, do you? Some had very thick, wiggly lips—others had hardly any lips at all. Some were very hairy and others were completely shaved. I tried to imagine what it would be like, posing for a magazine and having my pussy all over a centerfold, so that any man could look at it and masturbate over it.

"I gently played with my clitoris with my fingers. I think I was trying to postpone the moment when I would start using The Tongue. In the end, though, I switched on the television by using the remote control and put on the sex video with the sound very soft. There was kind of an introduction showing this girl in a teddy sitting on a bed, but the video got into the sex scenes pretty quickly. Two men came in and started talking to the girl and kissing her and fondling her breasts. The girl opened their jeans, took out their cocks and started to suck them, one after the other, in turn. I would never have watched anything like that before, but on that evening I *made* myself watch, to see how she did it. I noticed that she wasn't sucking their cocks so much as making love to them with her mouth . . . as if her mouth was a vagina. She licked them, too, especially around the heads of their cocks, and she kept poking the tip of her tongue into the little hole. And all the time she was masturbating them with her hand, quite hard.

"All of this oral sex turned me on so much that I switched on The Tongue to its lowest speed and ran it up and down between my legs. The feeling was incredible . . . it really made me shiver. I had never let Ted lick me before, but when I used The Tongue I could imagine what it felt like. Leastways, I *thought* I could—when he actually did it to me it was a hundred times sexier than The Tongue itself!

"I couldn't take my eyes off the video, the way she stretched her lips open so that these men could push their huge great purple cocks into her mouth . . . the way she kept rubbing them and digging her fingernails into their balls. I switched The Tongue on faster, and held it right up against my clitoris. I looked at myself in the mirror and I could see The Tongue going around and around and swirling my lips around. I couldn't believe how juicy my vagina was . . . I reached down with my other hand and smeared the juice all around my thighs. I felt as if I was doing something really bad. I mean, what if Ted could have seen me? But it was so exciting, you don't have any idea. I wasn't frightened anymore, and that's what made it even more exciting.

"In the video, the girl was licking both men at once, and rubbing their cocks so hard and fast that their balls were jiggling. Then one of them came—and shot sperm right into her mouth. She had her mouth wide open and her tongue out and he was squirting it onto her tongue. That shocked me, I have to tell you. But by then I was very aroused and even though it was a shock it was an exciting shock. I'd never seen a man come before—never seen the sperm actually shooting out of his cock. And I'd certainly never seen a woman swallowing it before. I guess what excited me more than anything was the expression on her face. Maybe she was only acting but she looked as if she was loving it. The other man came, too, and she had his sperm dripping down her chin. She didn't stop there, though. She went on kissing and sucking their cocks even though they were going soft.

"After that, there were scenes of another couple making love on the seashore. You could see the man's cock sliding in and out of the girl's vagina . . . and that made me feel like having a cock inside me, too. I opened up my vagina with my fingers and slid The Tongue up inside me, while the tongue was still waggling, and I carried on rubbing my clitoris with my other hand. The feeling I had between my legs, I can't tell you . . . it was like a burning tingle. It was almost too much to bear.

"I didn't have an orgasm that first time. I know it sounds silly, but I felt that masturbating myself all the way to orgasm would be like—well, being unfaithful. But I didn't really need an orgasm. What I'd done and what I'd seen had changed my attitude toward sex completely. I'd learned a whole lot about myself physically and emotionally. I'd learned to *enjoy* sexual feelings instead of being afraid of them. I'd seen how oral sex was done—and how exciting it could be. I felt like I'd made a fantastic discovery, like I was the first woman in the world to realize that sex wasn't threatening or frightening.

"I learned from the video that *words* aren't threatening, either. The girls kept saying things like 'Ram your cock into my cunt, baby,' and 'Shoot your load up my ass.' Before my self-discovery session I used to have a pet name for Ted's cock, which I'm far too embarrassed to tell you, and I would never say words like 'pussy' or 'cunt' or 'ass.' But what else can you call them? That's what they are—and when you say words like that when you're making love it turns you on all the more, doesn't it?

"When Ted climbed into bed that night he picked up his book from the nightstand and started to read. My heart was beating like a hammer, I can tell you. I was excited and frightened at the same time. I wanted him, and I wanted to please him, but I was still scared that I was going to do something wrong or that he wasn't going to like it.

"I turned over, slid my hand into the front of his pajamas, and took out his cock. He put down his book and looked at me and it was then that I thought everything was going to go wrong. But I started to fondle his cock and rub it up and down, the way the girl in the sex video had done, and he started to stiffen. He said, 'Mmmm, that's nice. What's gotten into you?'

"I said, 'Maybe I'm feeling hungry,' and I leaned over his cock and took the head of it into my mouth. Instantly he went even bigger and harder, and I had to stretch my mouth wide to get it all in. I rolled my tongue all the way around the head of his cock and sucked at his hole. All the time I kept on rubbing his shaft slowly up and down. You said in your book to grip it tight, and I did. All his veins bulged out and he was so hard that he felt as if he were carved out of ivory. To begin with he didn't say a word, but then he reached down and drew my hair back away from my face so that he had a clearer view of me sucking his cock, and he said, 'Oh, baby . . .' just like they did in that sex video. It was then that I was sure that I was doing it right.

"I took his cock as deep into my mouth as I could, sucking it and licking it and flicking it with the tip of my tongue. Once I started doing it, I found that oral sex almost came naturally—although there was one time when I sucked his cock too hard and hurt him. I had never kissed and played with a man's cock before, not like this, and I didn't want it to stop. I unbuttoned his pajamas and tugged them down to his knees. Then I licked his cock all the way down to his balls, and then I licked his balls, too, and gently took them into my mouth, one after the other. I licked around and around them until his pubic hair was all wet. Then I reached down and opened up the cheeks of his ass. There was his anus, all red, crinkled, and tight, surrounded by dark curly hair. I bent my head even further down and circled the tip of my tongue around it, around and around. He made a moaning kind of noise and he gripped my shoulders like he was drowning.

"I kissed his balls again and then I took his cock right in my mouth and started bobbing my head up and down just like the girl in the video. He was so tense that you would have thought that his backbone was going to snap. The fantastic thing was that I knew that he was close to coming, and that I was doing it to him. I could have stopped sucking him right then and he wouldn't have been able to do anything about it.

"He whispered, 'I'm coming,' and when I thought about it afterward I really appreciated it because he did give me the choice of whether I wanted to swallow his sperm or not. But I wanted it. I wanted to know what it tasted like. He suddenly said, 'Hah!' and my mouth was filled with this warm, sticky stuff. I don't know how to describe how it tasted. It wasn't exactly salty and it wasn't exactly sweet. It was a bit slithery, like egg white, but I swallowed it all the same, and then I sucked his cock so that I could swallow all the rest of it.

"I was so aroused by what I was doing that juice was literally dripping out of my pussy and sliding down my thighs. I turned over and lay on my back, and I opened my legs up wide. I began to masturbate myself, but Ted turned over, too, and knelt between my legs. He didn't try to stop me from masturbating but he joined in by licking my clitoris through the gaps between my fingers. I took my hand away and he licked me like The Tongue, only *his* tongue was much warmer and wetter and much more flexible. He licked me so beautifully that I almost screamed. It seemed like his tongue was everywhere—rolling around my clitoris, lapping around my vagina, poking into my anus.

"This time there wasn't any question of my not having an orgasm. He kept on licking me and licking me and I felt like I was dying and going to heaven. I could taste his sperm in my mouth. The funny things is, it's wet, but it makes your mouth feel quite dry. I thought about sucking his cock again so that I could swallow some more sperm and it was then that I climaxed.

"Afterward we lay side by side for a long time, holding each other, and we didn't say anything much. Then Ted propped himself up on his elbow and looked at me and said, "What happened to you? You were amazing. You never did anything like that before.' I think he was kind of suspicious that I might have met another guy. I said, 'I thought about what you said about me, that I just lie there in bed like I was dead, and I decided to come to life, that's all.'

"I went down on him again, and took his cock into my mouth. He was soft, but I love sucking his cock when it's soft, you can almost chew it. What's more, it doesn't take long before it starts to swell up again, and the next thing you know you're almost choking on it.

"For me, that day was just the beginning. Now we try all kinds of positions and all kinds of variations. Last week, while Ted was at work, I took a video of myself stripping and masturbating with all kinds of different objects. At the end of the video you can see me masturbating with two big cucumbers, one in my pussy and one up my anus, and then actually walking around the apartment naked with one of the cucumbers still poking out of my bottom. I showed it to Ted and we had the best night's sex ever.

"I guess you could say that the turning point for me was learning that sex isn't threatening at all. It's fun. It was when I saw that girl in the sex video *enjoying* herself. It was when I looked at myself and touched myself and masturbated with The Tongue. There's no harm in sex, nothing to be frightened of, only pleasure and affection. Before, I would have thought it was disgusting—even perverted—but I *enjoyed* walking around with a great big cucumber up my ass . . . nearly nine inches of it, fat and knobbly and *cool*, you know. It gives you such a sensation.

"I also learned that you have to show your partner that you want him. It's no good waiting for him to do it all."

Eloise wasn't completely to blame for the fact that her sex life with Ted was so mundane. Ted had a responsibility to find out why she was so reticent about trying sexual variations and then to educate and encourage her. He made a few tentative gestures, bringing home a sex video and some pornographic magazines (which, as it later turned out, proved to be invaluable), but it was obvious that he was afraid of upsetting Eloise and that he really didn't know how to coax her into trying more adventurous sex.

It was fortunate, therefore, that Eloise didn't simply sulk and say that her humdrum sex life was all Ted's fault and that he was the one who bore sole responsibility for doing something about it. She took her sexual destiny into her own hands and taught herself how to be sexually knowledgeable, sexually responsive, and sexually skillful. She trained herself not to be frightened or embarrassed by sex but to revel in all of its pleasures . . . and, as she said herself, if it gave her sexual pleasure to push a giant cucumber into her rectum, who can say that she was doing anything immoral or disgusting or antisocial? On the contrary, she was sexually liberated in the very best sense of the word, and her new willingness to experiment gave her pleasures that she had never dreamed of and a relationship with Ted that she willingly describes as "rock-solid."

Eloise said that overcoming her anxiety about sex was "one of the greatest experiences of my life." She realized that nothing that anybody does to enhance their sexual pleasure is immoral or "wrong," with the strict exception of acts that are performed against somebody else's will, or acts that endanger a person's health or safety.

Apart from a sparkling sex life with Ted, one of the side effects of her self-discovery has been that she finds herself much more socially confident and much more attractive to men in general. "It's something that happens inside of you. It's like you're much more sure of who you are. You're much more sure of your sexuality. I can be talking to a man at a party and I can think to myself, 'I know how to make you go wild in bed. I could suck your cock until you scream. I could ride on top of you until you think that you're in heaven. All the time, of course, I'm having this polite conversation and I know that I don't want anybody else but Ted. But knowing inside of yourself that you're a good lover gives you *power*, I think—and men can smell that power, like cats can smell catnip. It turns them on."

Sexual self-discovery can work equally well for women who currently don't have a partner. That inner confidence that Eloise was talking about can give them a lively aura to which men readily respond. Forget about *The Rules* and all that stuff about staying demure and dumb. Sally Jessy Raphael, the "Dear Abby of the Airwaves," rightly says that "when you exude warmth and self-confidence, you draw others toward you. Men and women often respond to each other from a gut level. The initial attraction process happens too fast for on-the-spot evaluation—it is automatic. This is why you must be in tune with your inner self and be comfortable with who you are. When you are able to do this, you will be relaxed and aware enough to be open to a man's romantic signals."

Many of the women who wrote to me and described their search for sexual self-discovery also mentioned that they were trying to discover themselves in many other ways, too. Some of them were trying to write poetry to express themselves. Others were interested in studying history or law or environmental conversation or charity work or any number of other subjects, from astronomy to zoology. Along with their burning interest in acquiring sexual knowledge and sexual expertise, they wanted to blossom intellectually, too.

There isn't any doubt in my mind that a woman who can show that she's educated, alert, and opinionated is much more attractive to today's man than a woman whose conversation is limited to what she saw on daytime TV yesterday afternoon. I don't mean that you have to be able to discuss Einstein's Theory of Relativity or the seasonal mating habits of the California grunion, but if you *do* have a developed interest in current affairs or music or any other subject that happens to appeal to you, you will always have something interesting to talk about and it will show men that you're very much more than just a hairstyle and a body and twenty lacquered nails. It will give you more social confidence, too. There is nobody more off-putting to a man than the girl who stands in the corner at parties looking as if all she has on her mind is whether she switched off the oven before she came out. He'll say, "Great party, isn't it?" and she'll say something like "Yes" or "I guess." Then there'll be a silence before he says something like "Do you want a drink?" and she'll say, "No, no thank you, I'm fine." Then there'll be an even longer silence before he says, "Are you friends of the X's (whoever is holding the party)?" and she'll say, "Yes." In the end, he won't bother asking any more questions. He'll say, "Excuse me," and go look for somebody more interesting.

What he'll be looking for is a girl who stands straight and looks men in the eye—a girl who smiles and laughs and *responds* when he approaches her. She'll willingly accept a drink—which gives him an errand to run on her behalf. She'll thank him kindly when he returns, and she'll immediately start to express an interest in who he is and what he does and what he thinks about the world. She won't be afraid to say what *she* thinks, either.

If she likes him, she'll use all of her feminine flirtatiousness to keep his attention—lowering her eyelashes, licking her lips, standing especially close to him. But at the same time she'll show him that she has depth and intelligence.

The Rules suggests that on a first date a woman shouldn't let a man know more than her name, college degree, and the number of siblings she has, but any woman who keeps as tight-lipped as that isn't being mysterious, she's being a pain—and she's drastically reducing her chances of forming one of those warm, immediate friendships that may very well lead to something more. Most men find women who play hard to get to be very frustrating—humiliating, even— and they'll very rarely persist if it looks as if starting up any kind of intimate relationship is going to be more trouble than it's worth.

Suzie, thirty-three, a divorcée from Boston, Massachusetts, told me, "One of my girlfriends said that I didn't attract men because I was always too open. She said i ought to pretend that I was unobtainable—that men would really have to work hard if they wanted to get me into bed. So when a man asked me for a date I always said no—the first time, anyway. I never let a man do anything more than kiss me on a first date, and I promised that I would never sleep with a man until I'd been dating him for at least three months. That was the theory. The reality was that if I said no the first time they asked me for a date they hardly ever tried again, and when I refused to sleep with a man after we'd been dating for more than a month, he said forget it and I never saw him again. *And* I really liked him."

Suzie went back to her old ways of being open and flirtatious and amusing, and within two months she was engaged to be married to a very good-looking doctor from a major Boston hospital.

There are no taboo topics when it comes to attracting men—provided you're always positive and upbeat. Maybe one exception is your previous husband or partner, especially if you're still carrying a major chip on your shoulder about him. Men like women with character but they don't like women with emotional baggage. The time for the deep and detailed sharing of your personal histories is after your relationship is very well established, and even then you should try to refrain from going into all the grisly details. As far as your new man is concerned, you're *his*, and he doesn't want to hear about your sex life with other men, no matter how inadequate they might have been.

Always be complimentary, rather than critical. Avoid running down your friends or your boss, and never say anything negative about your host or the party itself. Apart from the fact that it makes you sound downbeat, the man you're talking to may be very good friends with your hosts (or even, as one embarrassed woman discovered, your host's older brother). Let men know what you *do* like, rather than what you don't, and when he tells you about *his* interests, don't dismissively wrinkle up your nose. All right, so maybe you hate country music with a passion, but with the right partner maybe you could learn to like it just a little.

If he says, "Do you like Chinese food?" don't say, "Urgh," say, "I think I might if somebody could show me the right things to eat."

You don't have to act dumb. You don't have to hang

on his every word as if he were Moses freshly arrived from the mountain. You can be as witty and as warm as you like. The only point where I agree with *The Rules* wholeheartedly is when they advise against drinking too much. There is something uniquely embarrassing about a woman who is shrieking with laughter and can't quite manage to keep her balance.

You don't have to avoid politics or religion (except if you get *too* serious about it) and you certainly don't have to avoid sex. Discussing sex is one of the ways in which grown-up men and women flirt with each other, and it will give you an opportunity to show how confident and knowledgeable you are about it.

Of course *looking* attractive is crucial, and we've already discussed some of those special looks that men find particularly arousing. Men respond very much more to *visual* stimuli than women do. That's why they enjoy looking at the pictures in *Playboy* and *Hustler* and that's why they enjoy pornographic videos and strippers. A woman can look at a photograph of a naked man and it will hardly arouse her at all, but most men can look at a photograph of nothing more than a woman's vagina (without even seeing her face) and find it arousing enough to masturbate themselves to a climax.

Having said that, however, a man who is seriously looking for a long-term partner is looking for a woman who is not just arm candy but a real human being . . . a woman who can share his interests, and who has interests of her own that she is willing and able to share with him.

You should remember that most men are not the confident, decisive Romeos they pretend to be. Many men are very unsure of how to approach women and how to initiate a relationship. Yes—even those men who treat women as if they've been put on earth purely for men's amusement. In fact, *especially* those men who treat women like that. It's their way of protecting themselves in case they do or say anything gauche or embarrassing—and it disguises the fact that they're frightened of openly committing themselves. Quite often, the more they're attracted to you, the ruder and the more sexist they'll be. Don't be fooled by bluster or bantering. Once you have confidence in your own sexuality, you'll not only be highly attractive to almost any man who takes your fancy, you'll also be capable of putting him at ease—and then you'll be totally irresistible.

It may seem I have digressed from the topic of sexual self-discovery, but becoming sexually irresistible isn't simply a matter of sex. It's a matter of making the decision to develop your whole personality . . . of taking pride in your mind as well as your body. You wouldn't believe how many times I hear women saying, "I couldn't do that, I'm not clever enough"—or not skillful enough, or whatever. Not every woman can be a brilliant interior designer or an author or a painter or a research chemist. But every woman has some hidden talent, whether it's cookery or making jewelry or playing a musical instrument, and you owe it to yourself to develop it.

In fact you can develop it at the same time as your sexual talents, and the combination of doing both at once can give tremendous added excitement to both.

Many of the women who successfully tried my sexual self-discovery sessions wrote to say that they would have liked to be able to carry them a stage further. Could I suggest a longer session, maybe, with the inclusion of more sexual experimentation?

For that reason I devised an All-Day Self-Pleasuring

Plan. It will not only give you hours of opportunity to try out new erotic variations at your leisure, but it will give you the time to interweave your sexual self-loving with some of your nonsexual self-development. You don't have to have a partner to try out the All-Day Plan, but if you do, it's also intended to have you in a high state of sexual readiness by the time you meet your man at the end of the day.

You'll have to make some preparations for your All-Day Plan. First of all, of course, you'll have to earmark a day when you know that you're going to be completely alone and undisturbed—and these days, that isn't always easy. One woman simply told her boss that she was sick and took a whole day off work. Another managed to persuade her husband to take the children to a theme park. If you have to invent some outrageous excuse, don't start getting a conscience about it. This is going to be *your* day, for *your* benefit, and the man in your life is going to benefit, too . . . even if you haven't found him yet. Actually, the secrecy of sneaking an illicit day off can add to its excitement.

Once you've picked a day, make some plans for how you're going to spend it, and gather together everything you're going to need. Sexually, you should have at least one penis-shaped vibrator or dildo, although I recommend two—one of them for vaginal stimulation and one for anal stimulation. It's more hygienic to have two, and you will be able to stimulate yourself vaginally and anally at the same time. There are plenty of reputable mail-order companies who will send you catalogs of sex aids, so that you can choose what you want at your leisure. You may want to select a thinner vibrator for anal stimulation . . . some of them are not much more than flexible rubbery wands with knobs on them. But if you're interested in having anal intercourse with your partner you should buy one that's at least as big as a man's erect member. As a guideline, the average American male has a penis 6.375 inches long and 4.12 inches in girth.

You might like to select some other sex toys, too, apart from vibrators. During your All-Day Plan you'll have plenty of time to try different clothing and devices. Try to choose at least one kind of stimulator that you can wear while you're walking around . . . such as a butterfly vibrator. This is a butterfly-shaped "buzzer" that you can attach by straps to your clitoral area, and which will give you constant stimulation for as long as you want it. Another good All-Day aid is orgasm pants, which are tight latex pants with a vibrator fixed inside them. You pull on the pants, sliding the vibrator into your vagina as you do so, and there it stays, vibrating away, until you decide to take your pants off again. I've talked to several girls who like to wear these under their clothes when they go to work—"My boss couldn't understand why I spent the whole day smiling."

You could even go to the expensive lengths of buying yourself a whole man. The cheapest are inflatable, with vibrating penises attached between their legs. A German company produces a luxury version in lifelike latex, complete with erect penis, scrotum, and anal access, but the last time I saw one advertised it was well over fifteen hundred dollars.

Buy some condoms, too, of any variety that tickle your fancy. If you're going looking for a new partner, or if you're not one hundred percent satisfied that your current partner doesn't carry the HIV virus, then condoms are obviously essential. Also, it's wiser to use a condom if you and your partner are thinking about anal sex—his penis may *look* perfectly clean when it comes out of your anus, but as I said before, the rectum harbors some very virulent bacteria, and there's a risk that he may develop a urethral infection, particularly if he's been pushing himself into you very hard. If you use a condom you can go straight from anal sex to vaginal sex without the need to halt the proceedings while he goes off to the bathroom to wash himself.

Incidentally, recent reports have indicated that more and more women are risking sexual intercourse without condoms. Quite apart from the consequences of an unwanted pregnancy, the danger of contracting AIDS is just as high as it always was, so do make sure that you always keep condoms handy when you're going to a party or a dinner-dance or any social function where you might find that your eyes meet the eyes of a handsome stranger and one thing leads to another. It does happen—and it's much more likely to happen if you're sexually irresistible. And always keep a selection of condoms by the bed. These days they come in such kaleidoscopic colors and flavors that a dish of assorted rubbers on the nightstand looks almost good enough to eat.

The sexually irresistible woman doesn't regard it as an interruption when her lover fits on a condom. She includes it as part of her sex play—either by rolling it on by hand, or better still by using her mouth. New York sex counselor Patti Britton, Ph.D., says, "I love to do it with my mouth . . . It fulfills one of the man's favorite things, which is oral sex, plus it's fun for the woman."

You can buy condoms in mint, strawberry, chocolate, and bubble-gum flavors—and many more—or you can customize a plain condom by smothering it in your own favorite sauce or syrup. Jaynie, a twenty-four-year-old shoestore assistant from Chicago, Illinois, told me that she loved sucking her boyfriend's condom-clad penis when it was smothered in red currant jelly—"His balls, too!"

Other varieties of condoms have prongs or ribs or hard little latex nubs for increased sensation. One, the Pleasure Plus, has a large pouch on the end that loosely rolls and unrolls while you and your partner make love, giving you the feeling that he has a very large foreskin. You can also buy condoms that glow in the dark, and polyurethane condoms that warm up to body temperature.

A few items of erotic clothing will add to your pleasure, too. Maybe you've never thought of yourself as the kind of woman who would wear a quarter-cup bra or open-crotch panties, or parade around the house wearing nothing but black stockings and a garter belt. But you never know what excitement you may get from it until you try. Your all-day pleasurefest is intended to give you a complete break from routine, from rules, and from doing things a certain way just because you've always done them that way. This is a day for you to discover yourself—to find out what excites you, both physically and mentally.

If you can obtain one or two erotic videos or a sexy magazine, so much the better—but they're not essential. Most of your pleasure will be happening inside your mind. However, do make an effort to get hold of a video camera—or, failing that, an ordinary camera with a delay timer on it so that you can take photographs of yourself.

In the morning, once you're alone, your self-pleasuring can begin. Relax as much as you can. Keep on reminding yourself that every minute of this day is entirely for you, to calm yourself and find yourself. It's a day to develop the very sensual and attractive person that you are—so that not only are *you* aware that you're one of the most sexually irresistible women you've ever met, *he'll* be aware of it, too—even if you haven't found him yet.

Lie in bed for at least an hour longer than you normally do, indulging yourself with coffee, orange juice, and fresh fruit. Watch TV if you want to, or play some music. There's just one stipulation: you should be naked, and you'll be staying more or less naked for the rest of the day.

As you lie there, think about all the things that you'd like to do in bed, but never have, either because you were too inhibited to tell your partner, or because you didn't have a partner with whom you could do them. Mentally leaf through your sexual fantasies—even the most extreme ones—and make a note of which ones arouse you the most.

At the same time, massage your breasts and your nipples, using a little body lotion or massage oil, and then gradually slide your hands down between your legs and slowly stimulate yourself with your fingers. Do it very gently, just to get yourself into the mood. Use a hand mirror to watch yourself as you're doing it. As in the shorter self-discovery session, you should take some time to become familiar with your vulva and its anatomy, and what kind of fingering gives you the most pleasure.

Four different women described their sexual yearnings to me and I prescribed an all-day session of sexual discovery in order to see how successful they would then be in fulfilling them.

Ella is a twenty-six-year-old dental nurse from Minneapolis, Minnesota. She's blonde and extremely pretty, and she was never short of boyfriends. "All my classmates were so jealous, but they needn't have been. I dated all of the good-looking guys . . . the captain of the athletics team, the college football hero. But they were all so into themselves. They didn't have any idea how to satisfy a woman, and I don't suppose they've learned how to do it, even now."

Ella never had what she considered a truly fulfilling sexual relationship. While she found it easy to attract men, she found it almost impossible to attract the kind of man that she really wanted. "Most guys treat me like a trophy, and they never seem to understand that I have feelings and needs of my own." Although she had had seven affairs by the time she was twenty-five, she had never achieved a real orgasm except by masturbation. "The guys always came first. I mean, sometimes they came as soon as they put their cock in. So what could I do? I faked it. It got to the point where I never even tried to reach a climax. I just let them do it and then I screamed and shook and said *oh-oh-oh* and all that kind of stuff and they *loved* it. Like they'd never made a girl actually *scream* before. But for me it was nothing. It was like reading a really exciting book and finding the last four pages missing."

Ella enjoyed lovemaking (and why not?) but she simply didn't know how to take control of her sexual relationships so that she could get out of them the satisfaction she so badly needed. "I love sex. I love men. But they always leave me feeling so frustrated. Sometimes I think that there's something wrong with me." Her frustration inevitably led to her relationships breaking down, and having to initiate yet another search for Mr. Right.

Ella's story is typical of thousands of women all across the country, and it goes to show that pretty girls don't necessarily have more fun than ordinary-looking girls. In fact they tend to be a magnet for the kind of man who regards a girl as a fashion accessory rather than a human being—vain, arrogant men who believe that they're world-class studs when in fact they're usually world-class duds. Let's be realistic: there will always be women who are attracted to a man's wallet rather than his looks or his sexual prowess. I've frequented nightclubs and gaming clubs and there are always rich, ugly men with beautiful young girls hanging on their arms. This isn't an indictment of women in general, but it does happen. Money and power are very sexually arousing. But on the whole, these girls don't get much more than a temporary entrée to the world of glamour and wealth. They rarely get sexual satisfaction, and they rarely know *how* to get it. But there is a way to attract the men you really want, and once you've started a sexual relationship, there are plenty of ways in which you can improve their lovemaking so that they satisfy you every single time.

Apart from finding a man who could bring her to orgasm, Ella's recurring fantasy was to make love in the great outdoors. "I've always fantasized about having sex in the woods someplace, or maybe in a field. I've never done it, and I've never had the nerve to suggest it, but wouldn't it be great?"

She felt that, outdoors, she could be more herself, and that she would have more sexual confidence. "I know that I have a good figure. I'd feel really happy, running around naked in the open air. I'd feel free." Although she didn't know it, she was looking for a sexual environment in which she could feel as if she were in control. Although it is hardly ever discussed in books about sex, *where* you make love is one of the most important factors in enhancing your sexual relationships. I'm not just talking about sexual intercourse on the kitchen table, for the sake of a little variety. I'm talking about making love where *you* feel stimulated, where *you* feel aroused, and where *you* can call the shots.

Jean, a twenty-seven-year-old illustrator for an advertising agency in Madison, Wisconsin, said, "Brett and I first made love after the agency's Christmas party. We went to a motel and made love all night and it was great! The first few nights we spent together were great. But then he kept taking me off to the same motel and I began to think, is this it? We're going to spend year after year making love in the same motel? Men just don't have any imagination, do they? They think that if something was great once, it's always going to be great, no matter how many times you do it.

"We were at work one day and I met Brett in the corridor just outside the ladies' room. I don't know why I did it, but I took hold of his hand and pulled him right in through the door. He kept saying, "No, no, I shouldn't be in here! What if somebody sees us?' But I kept on kissing him and fondling him and I dragged him into one of the cubicles and closed the door.

"He said, 'This is crazy! If I get caught in here they'll fire me!' But I wasn't going to have him backing out now. I unbuttoned my blouse and took off my bra. Then I unzipped my skirt and took that off, too, and stepped right out of my pantyhose, so that I was completely naked.

"Brett was going out of his mind, but I was turning him on, too. Well, I could tell that by the bulge in his pants. I sat down on the john and I opened my legs up wide. I'd only just gone for a bikini wax, so my cunt was completely smooth and bare. I said, 'Come on . . . touch me. You like touching me, don't you?' He bent over and kissed me, and fondled my breasts, and then he ran his hand down between my legs.

"At that moment, the bathroom door opened and two of my colleagues came in and started talking to each other. One of them came right into the next cubicle and we could hear her sit down and start pissing. I opened up Brett's pants and took out his cock and it was enormous. The head was all purple and he was so stiff that he actually curved upward. I held his cock in my hand and squeezed it hard. Then I kissed it and licked it and took it into my mouth. All the time my colleagues were still talking and they were only inches away from us—but there I was with Brett's cock in my mouth, sucking him and poking my tongue into his little hole.

"He kept on stroking the lips of my cunt and playing with my clitoris. Then he slid his middle finger right up my hole. It felt so gorgeous that it was all I could do to stop myself from moaning out loud. I unbuckled his belt and pulled his pants halfway down his thighs. I loved his thighs—they were muscular and suntanned with all this fine blonde hair. His pubic hair was blonde, too. I took hold of his balls in both hands and kept on sucking and sucking, as deep as I could. I wanted to swallow him up.

"He was kissing the top of my head and running his hand through my hair, tugging it and pulling it, but with his other hand he was pushing his finger in and out of my cunt. Then he pushed in another finger, and another, and I made a noise—like *unnhh!*—even though I had my mouth full of cock. The girl in the next cubicle called out, 'Jean—is that you?' and I was so nervous and excited that I started pissing. I couldn't stop myself. I pissed right into Brett's hand, all over his fingers, but he didn't mind at all. In fact it turned him on more than ever. He held his hand right in the stream of piss and he massaged my cunt at the same time, all around it, so that I was all wet.

"I took his cock out of my mouth and stood up. I bent over the toilet, holding on to the seat, and he opened up my cunt with his fingers and pushed himself into me, all the way up, all the way up to the balls. I could feel every single inch of him, his cock was so big and warm, and his balls were thumping against my cunt lips. My friend called 'Jean—are you all right?' but I couldn't even answer. Brent was fucking me so hard, and there was such a strong smell of piss and sex. It was all so dirty and so dangerous! And of course it was different, too. Not like that same old motel room.

"I don't know how I managed it, but I actually had an orgasm, bent double over the toilet. Brett kept on going for a little while longer, but then he climaxed, too. That was the first time I ever really *felt* a man's sperm shoot up inside me. . . . We stood there holding each other tight for who knows how long. His cock was softer, but it was still quite big, and smothered in sperm. I knelt down on the floor and sucked it for him, that lovely salty-dry taste of sperm, but mixed with my taste, too. I don't think that anything in the world tastes as sexy as a man's and a woman's juices, mixed. What you might call a cocktail of love, yes?

"I don't know if anybody found out what we'd been doing in the ladies' room, but it made all the difference to our relationship. From then on, we fucked almost anyplace. We didn't need to go to a motel. I used to go into Brett's office, open his pants, take out his cock, and give it a long, lingering suck before zipping him up and walking out like nothing had happened. If we were alone together in an elevator, he pulled up my skirt in the back and pulled down my pantyhose and pushed his fingers up my cunt. Then, if the elevator stopped at the next floor, he would stand on the other side of the car and very nonchalantly sniff and suck his finger, and smile at me. Like after what we did in the bathroom, Brett entered into the game, and made it even more exciting. But I had to do something first— something to get us out of a rut."

Barbara is a thirty-one-year-old cosmetician from Tallahassee, Florida. She married at the age of twenty-two, had two children, a boy and a girl, but her marriage broke up after her husband lost his job and started drinking. She calls the last two years of her marriage "the black years"—but, determined to make a new start, she joined local clubs and associations and played a vital part in fund-raising for local charities. Her problem? "Men seem to be attracted to me, but when they find out that I'm a divorcée with two children to take care of, they back off. They seem to think that I'm carrying too much baggage, you know? These days, men don't seem to be prepared to make any kind of commitment. I'm not necessarily looking for another husband. I'd be happy with a man friend who took me out from time to time and took me to bed from time to time. When you're young, you never think that you're going to have a life without sex. But I'm only thirty-one, and that's what's happened to me."

Barbara's fantasy was surprisingly extreme, and it took a long time for me to cajole her into telling me what it was. "If you really want to know, I'd like to be tied up, and blindfolded, have two or three men in the room—maybe even four or five. They can do what they like with me, and I won't be able to stop them.

They can fuck me, one after the other. They can fuck me at the same time, if they want to. They can push things up my pussy or into my asshole—candles or vibrators or toilet brush handles. They can rub their cocks up against my face and sit on top of me so that I have to lick their asses. They can force their cocks and their balls into my mouth. They can spank me. They can call me anything they like—whore, bitch, cunt. They can masturbate all over me."

Let me say right away that Barbara wasn't a masochist—somebody who can derive sexual satisfaction *only* out of being abused or humiliated. But during "the black years" it had been up to her to her to keep her family together, both financially and emotionally, and her ex-husband had accused her again and again of being domineering. At the end of the marriage, she was exhausted from shouldering all of the family's responsibilities, and tired of making all the decisions. Quite simply, she wanted to feel helpless again.

She didn't *really* want to be sexually assaulted in the way she described in her fantasy, but she did want a sexual partner or partners who would be virile and decisive and drag *her* into the bedroom instead of the other way around.

You should remember that fantasies are fantasies, and nothing more—and that during sexual excitement the most respectable woman can have the most outrageous erotic ideas. Often these ideas are so extreme that she won't ever mention them to anyone else, not even her partner. But as I say, they are nothing more than one way your imagination serves to increase your sexual arousal, and as such you should welcome them and encourage them rather than feel ashamed of them. For instance, rape is an abominable crime and no woman would find it arousing if it really happened, but *fantasies* of rape are extremely common. So are fantasies of bondage and sexual mistreatment such as whipping and spanking and being forced to commit oral sex.

Other common masochist fantasies include being stripped in public (such as being a slave in a slave market) and being raped and abused in extremely filthy surroundings.

If you've ever had a really "dirty" fantasy . . . or if you still do, frequently or infrequently, you have absolutely nothing to worry about. What happens inside your head is your business, and nobody was ever hurt by a fantasy unless they took the chance of acting out something very extreme for real. Most of the time fantasies are far more exciting if that's what they stay—fantasies.

Linda is a forty-two-year-old magazine editor from San Francisco, California. She's five feet four, with blonde curls, a well-boned face, and, "Yes, I inherited my mother's breasts; they're much too big for me." During her early twenties, Linda worked as a legal secretary, and she was married at the age of twenty-six to a very busy and successful lawyer. However, it only took a few months for her to realize that she'd made a serious mistake. "Dean was hardly ever home, and when he *was* home he was always on the phone to his clients or going through paperwork or playing golf. He used to bring me flowers and he never forgot a birthday or an anniversary, but that was only because he had a very efficient secretary. I realized that he couldn't see any further than my face and my breasts. I was an acquisition, not a human being. If I ever said anything about politics or science or anything serious he would look at me in amazement, like his pet cat had suddenly learned to talk."

Linda and her husband were divorced after a little over four years, but it didn't take Linda long to realize that a twenty-six-year-old single secretary with a sassy smile may be irresistible to men, but the mating game is very different for a thirty-one-year-old divorcée with no job to go to.

"I was only thirty-one, but I felt like I was an old maid. My friends and neighbors never invited me to dinner parties anymore because they thought their husbands were going to go after me. I tried singles bars but I never met anybody there except divorced men who were feeling just as down and unwanted as I was, and that was the last thing I needed. I went through eighteen months of loneliness and depression, and in the end I was taking so many pills that I practically rattled.

"I went to a shrink for four or five years. She kept me sane, but she didn't find me what I really needed, which was a partner. A man companion, maybe a husband. Was that too much to ask? Anyhow, I did what you suggested, which was to turn my attention to my whole self, and not worry exclusively about sex. That's when I took the journalism course and got the job on the magazine. At least I had pride in what I was doing. But I still didn't feel attractive to men. I did all the things you're supposed to do. I laughed at their jokes. I looked them in the eye. But in the end they always turned away from me as if I didn't exist, and I was beginning to think that my husband might have been right, and I *didn't* really exist—not as a person who was worth knowing, anyway.

"About two months ago, though, I was invited to a tennis party by some friends of my parents. I was teamed up in the doubles with a young man about half my age. His name was Peter, and he was practically a demigod, believe me. He was tall and suntanned, with perfect teeth, and he was super-fit. With him, I played the most strenuous game of tennis I'd played since high school. And while I was playing, I suddenly realized that I wasn't trying so hard because he was good. I was trying to impress him. I was trying to attract him. And he was only twenty-two!

"He seemed to like me, and he spent a long time talking to me and asking me questions, because he was thinking of going into media, too. I made an effort not to patronize him—not to treat him like a kid, and I think he appreciated it. But I don't know whether he thought of me as a potential lover.

"Afterward, I went into the house to shower. The downstairs shower was occupied so I went upstairs. As I walked along the landing I saw that the bathroom door was a little bit open. I was about to go inside when I saw that Peter was in there, standing in front of the mirror, toweling his hair. He was completely naked.

"I should have turned around and gone back downstairs, but I just stood and stared. He had these amazing sculptured muscles, a totally flat stomach, and narrow hips. His ass was tight and rounded, and completely tanned, too, so he must have been in the habit of sunbathing in the nude. His cock was huge, and because it kept bobbing against the side of the sink, it was half erect. The head was a beautiful pale purple, but the rest of his cock was tanned with a dark vein running through it. His pubic hair was long and dark and very silky.

"His cock stiffened even more until it was poking upward. I could hardly breathe. At that moment there was nothing more I wanted in the world than to have that cock inside my cunt, and his pubic hair to be tangling with mine. But then I caught sight of myself in the mirror and I thought, 'Linda, what the hell are you doing?' and I quietly turned around and went away. I was so ashamed of myself my cheeks were burning.

"But that night I lay awake almost all night, thinking what it would be like to have a much younger man for a lover. I kept picturing Peter's body, and that enormous cock. It rose up so hard and so tight it almost touched his belly button. I fantasized about him carrying me into my bedroom, lifting up my tennis skirt, and taking down my panties. I fantasized about it and I could almost *feel* it, you know? His lean suntanned body on top of mine, and that huge long cock pushing into my cunt. I put my hand between my legs to masturbate and I found that I was wetter than I'd ever been. So I thought to myself, maybe I *do* need a younger man, somebody like Peter . . . but how does a woman like me go about finding a younger man and starting up a sexual relationship with him without making a fool of herself?"

In the twenty-five years that I have been counseling men and women who have had difficulty in finding a fulfilling sexual relationship, I have come across many instances of older women having their sexual confidence restored by starting an affair with a younger man. The benefits work both ways: an older woman is usually much more sexually experienced and less inhibited than the girls that the younger man is accustomed to dating. She knows what she needs, and she can teach him timing and technique and many sexual variations that he hasn't yet tried. Jeff, twenty-one, a student from Milwaukee, Wisconsin, had a seven-month relationship with forty-four-year-old Pamela

Sue, who worked at his local library. "I knew about anal intercourse, for sure. It was one of those things the guys talked about at college. But one night, when we were together, Pamela Sue turned her back on me, took hold of my cock, and guided it into her asshole. It was incredible. I pushed my cock into her all the way up to my balls and she didn't even flinch. It was just like somebody with a warm hand, gripping my cock really tight, and when she rippled her muscles, that was something else. The only trouble was, I climaxed right there and then, I couldn't help it, and filled up her asshole with come. But the next time she showed me how to do it slower, and not to get so excited." The next time was less than an hour later, and this is one of the advantages for older women having affairs with younger men. Young men in their twenties will have far more sexual stamina than men in their forties and fifties; and will do a great deal to restore a woman's belief in her own attractiveness. Which—as we've seen—is one of the keys to being sexually irresistible.

Lastly, here's Nancy, a twenty-seven-year-old bank executive from Memphis, Tennessee, with a bright career future ahead of her. Nancy's problem is that she has trouble keeping her weight down and she admits that she has "absolutely no confidence" when it comes to men. Since leaving high school she has had only two serious boyfriends—both of whom were generous-spirited and supportive, but neither of whom came anywhere close to being the kind of man that Nancy fantasizes about.

"I don't want a kind, friendly, overweight guy, which is all I've had so far. I want a thin, mean, good-looking guy—a guy who's going to give me a hard time if I pig out. I'm sexy. I *know* I'm sexy. I haven't fucked very often but when I did I loved it. I could give any guy a truly fantastic time in bed if only I had the chance. If he wanted me to suck his cock I promise that I'd suck it all night. But every day I get up and look at myself in the mirror and I'm still a hundred and forty pounds and my stomach's still sticking out and my breasts are still enormous and I still have to wear the same glasses. Sometimes I feel that life is so unfair. I mean, when they were handing out the terrific looks, why didn't *I* get any?"

Nancy's plea is echoed by thousands of women all across the country. They have strong sexual feelings, and they are perfectly capable of being wonderful lovers. But genetics have denied them the facial bone structure and the tip-tilted nose and the pouting lips that are regarded in the United States as classical good looks. Instead of *Baywatch*-style figures, they have bulges and bumps and all the oddities that flesh can be heir to.

Well, here's the news. There is a way that you can make yourself over so that you can be irresistible to men, no matter what your weight. That's not to say that you shouldn't make every effort to control your diet. If you're slimmer, you'll be healthier and much more active and perhaps a better lover in bed.

What you can do is to introduce your dieting as part of your All-Day Self-Pleasuring Session . . . make it a *part* of your sexual pleasure, make it a *part* of what you intend to be. No matter what they promise ("Drop a Dress Size in Three Days!"), the fact is that diet plans never work and will always end up making you feel depressed and defeated, and will probably lead to you eating more and becoming even *more* overweight. All diet plans are published for the enrichment of their authors and publishers and not because they will have any significant effect on your weight or the shape of your body.

Only one diet plan has ever been proven to be effective, and that is to eat fewer calories than you usually use up in your daily activity, and you will gradually and safely lose weight. That's all. It doesn't matter *what* you eat. You can eat a big slice of chocolate cake if you want to—provided your total daily intake doesn't exceed the total amount you usually use up.

Think of yourself as that speeding train in the old Laurel and Hardy movie, where they're having to chop up the passenger cars to provide fuel for the locomotive's boiler. The boiler burned the wood, the train got smaller. If they'd kept adding on more cars faster than they burned them, the train would have gone on growing bigger. If you burn up just a few more calories a day than you usually ingest, *and you keep it up over a period of time*, then you'll be amazed how much you lose. A little controlled exercise, a little less food. It doesn't have to be agony. And don't worry if it seems to take forever. The New You will be waiting for you, in the mirror, in six months' time.

Meanwhile, let's try something that will bring you almost *immediate* results—an All-Day Self-Pleasuring Session that will give you much more sexual confidence than you've ever had before. It worked—in different ways, and in varying degrees—with each of my four volunteers, and I don't have any doubt at all that it could work for you. Not only will you become much more tempting to the man in your life, you'll experience hours of self-indulgent sexual pleasure.

Many women have written to me and said, "I feel very guilty if I masturbate. It's almost like being unfaithful" or "Masturbating makes me feel like I've given up hope of ever finding a partner" or "I was brought up to believe that touching themselves is something that nice girls just don't do."

However, all modern therapists agree that any sexual pleasure is good for your physical and mental well-being. Sexually satisfied women are better balanced socially: more sure of themselves, more successful, more friendly, more progressive. And it makes very little difference if they derive their sexual satisfaction from intercourse with a partner or from masturbation. Feeling the urge to masturbate is nothing to feel guilty about, even if you're married or currently involved in a long-term sexual relationship. You can't commit adultery with your own fingers. Masturbating shows that you have a normal sex drive, just like most other women. When you feel like doing it, do it. Regardless of dire Victorian warnings that masturbators would become hopeless idiots or grow hair on the palms of their hands, masturbation is one of the few really pleasant experiences in life that can be achieved without any kind of physical or mental risk.

Sheila, twenty, a factory worker from Seattle, Washington, wrote me that she masturbated every time she felt the urgent need for ice cream. "I kind of traded one treat for another. I lost so much weight and all of my friends said that I really glow. I don't have a man yet but I'm looking much sexier and I'm feeling much sexier . . . I'd recommend it to anyone."

Swapping ice cream for sexual self-pleasuring may seem like a very small change to make in your life. Yet for Sheila it was a very dramatic step to take. It meant that she had consciously decided that when she felt the need for emotional comfort, she wasn't going to be negative and go looking for it in a bucket of Rocky Road. She was going to be positive, and seek it in sexual orgasm.

"I've taught myself to climax more quickly. I do this by squeezing my thighs together and flipping the tip of my clitoris very fast. I've also taught myself to hold off an orgasm so that the pleasuring seems to go on forever. I open my legs wide and rub the shaft of my clitoris very gently and very slowly. I'll tell you, by the time I find myself a man, I'm going to be able to give him the time of his life."

Apart from that, Sheila said, "For the first time in a long time, I feel happy. I'm losing weight, and I'm getting all the sex that I can find time for."

Now let's continue with your All-Day Self-Pleasuring Session. You've bathed or showered; you've dried yourself. You're alone in your house or apartment, with nobody to disturb you. This is the time you should affirm (out loud if you like) that this day is yours. *This is the day on which I will discover myself . . . my mind and my body. This is the day on which I will learn to put all sexual embarrassment behind me, forever. This is the day on which I will explore my wildest fantasies but also my real, day-to-day needs. I will look back on this day in years to come and remember it—because it is the day on which I sexually empowered myself. As an individual. As a person with her own opinions and her own tastes and her own sexual desires. As the most irresistible woman that the men in my life are ever going to meet.*

CHAPTER FIVE

How to Get in Touch with Your Sexual Self

"I've never spent a whole day just *indulging* myself before," said Ella. "I have to tell you that I'm feeling kind of guilty about it."

"I'm not sure that I can walk around naked," said Nancy. "I know there won't be anybody around except me, but I'm very self-conscious about the way I look."

Barbara admitted to being "nervous . . . especially about really extreme masturbation—you know, with different objects."

Linda said, "Self-pleasuring seems kind of incomplete . . . you know, like going to a restaurant and eating a meal on your own with a book propped up against the catsup bottle."

However, your All-Day Session won't be like that at all. Unlike eating alone in a restaurant, you'll be meeting someone, and getting to know them well: your own sexual personality. This is a time for you to discover what you can do for the men in your life, and what you want the men in your life to do for you.

Let's flash forward to what Ella said at the *end* of her All-Day Session. "I think the most important thing I learned was about *attitude*, you know? Up until now,

I'd always kind of assumed that when it came to sex, it was the man who was supposed to be in charge. But a man can't possibly know how to arouse you if you don't take some of the responsibility for yourself.

"Another thing I learned was how much men like you to suck and play with their cocks. I've fondled and kissed a guy's cock once or twice, but I've never been sure whether men like it or not. But I read what you said about oral sex, and I watched two or three porno movies, and now I can't wait to have my mouth filled up with a big hard cock.

"I love the bit where you say that you should think strongly sexual thoughts when you meet a man you like. One of the partners in my dental practice is so gorgeous. I can't wait to see him Monday and talk to him about dental implants, while all the while I'm thinking to myself, 'If only you knew what I could do for you if I opened up your pants and took your cock out. I'd chew your big fat purple head till you screamed!' I love that. I think it's going to work."

Ella pretty much summed up the whole philosophy of an All-Day Self-Pleasuring Session. Once you're sexually confident . . . once you can dare to think of the things that you'd like a man to do for you, or the things that you'd like to do to him . . . you'll acquire an indefinable aura of sexuality.

After you've spent some pleasant, leisurely time in bed, your All-Day Self-Pleasuring Session should continue with a shower or a bath—for which you should have bought yourself a new and expensive shower gel or bath foam. Make a point of spending twice as long in the bath or the shower as you usually do. Massage your neck and your shoulders with soap, then spend as long as you like massaging your breasts and your nipples. Lie back in the bath and close your eyes and think of the man you'd really like to make love to you—whether it's your partner or a movie star who takes your fancy or a completely imaginary man altogether, like the character Antonio in the story *Artists and Models* by the celebrated female erotic writer Anaïs Nin: "He had a golden brown body, a penis as smooth as the rest of his body, big, firm as a polished wooden baton. She fell on him and took it into her mouth. His fingers went everywhere, into her anus, into her sex; his tongue, into her mouth, into her ears."

As you lie in the bath, think of what you could do to excite and please the man in your life—or the man that you'd like to have in your life. Keep on massaging yourself as you do so, and before the water begins to turn cold, massage yourself between your legs, play with your clitoris and your vagina. If you've been able to find yourself a waterproof vibrator, this is a wonderful time to use it, but a solid dildo is almost as good. (On no account, though, use an electric vibrator in the bath!)

This is a time to relax, and to drift. Whatever anxieties you've been having about sex and your sexual relationships (or your *lack* of sexual relationships), let them slide away. For the next few hours you're going to be living in a world of your own where you can have any kind of sex you want. By the end of the day you should have both the attitude and the ability to change your love life forever.

While you're in the bath, you might want to shave off or trim your pubic hair. This is one of those sexual variations that arouses men intensely, although few of them will admit to it. If you were to ask the man in your life if you should shave yourself bare down there, he would probably shrug and say, "It's up to you." He's right, too. It *is* up to you. That's what makes it so erotic for him if you do . . . you've deliberately chosen to expose the most private part of your body for his personal pleasure.

You can remove pubic hair with a razor or a combination of razor and bikini-line depilatory cream, or you can have it waxed. Electrolysis will remove pubic hair permanently, but that might not be a good idea since you may want to grow it back in the future.

Of course, you don't have to remove all of it. Kathy, a twenty-two-year-old Titian-haired bookstore assistant from Indianapolis, Indiana, said, "I like to have a bare, hair-free cunt. But at the same time I do like my boyfriends to know that I'm a genuine redhead. So I always leave just a little tuft right above my clitoris. I guess it gives them a tickle, too!"

You can shave your hair into a heart shape or a star shape. I've even seen lightning bolts and sun rays. But whatever you do, it's an explicit statement to your partner that you've done it for his sexual excitement.

Renata, a twenty-four-year-old receptionist from New York, shaved off all her pubic hair for a two-week vacation in Fort Lauderdale, Florida, and the effect on her boyfriend was electrifying. "Brad and I had booked the vacation in the hope that we could straighten things out between us. We'd been arguing a whole lot. Most of the time I didn't even know what we were arguing about. But our sex life wasn't very good, either. Brad was working such long hours that he was too tired for lovemaking in the evening, and if he managed to make it in the morning he was always in a rush. I felt that he was taking me for granted, you know? I was supposed to be his lover, not just the girl who cooked his meals and took care of his laundry. He could have had a housekeeper to do that.

"Anyhow, we went down to Fort Lauderdale and of

course I shaved my cunt because I was going to be wearing a bikini most of the time. At first I left a bit of hair in the middle, but I thought it looked stupid so I shaved it all off. I liked it, sure. In fact I liked it a lot. I think women look beautiful with bare cunts; you can see everything.

"We reached the hotel and unpacked our suitcases, and Brad said, 'Let's go for a swim.' He undressed first. I had my back to him but I was undressing in front of the closet, which had all of these mirrored doors. He was just about to step into his shorts when he turned around and saw me. He didn't say a word, but you should have seen his face! He came toward me and with every step he took his cock grew bigger. By the time he reached me it was standing up totally stiff. He put his arms around me and held my breasts. Then he slid one hand down my stomach and touched me between my legs.

"He said, 'What a turn-on! When did you do that?'

"I said, 'You like it?'

"And he said, 'I think Christmas has come early!'

"So I said, 'Just so long as *you* don't!' Pretty good joke, huh? But it almost happened. He turned me around and took me in his arms and kissed me, and his cock was so hard that it was pressing against my stomach. I took hold of it and squeezed it and circled my thumb around the top of it and it was all wet and slippery already.

"Brad lifted me up and carried me over to the bed. He lay me down and opened my legs, and he looked at my cunt as if it was the Holy Grail or something. He took his cock in his hand and rubbed it all around my bare cunt lips. He rolled it from side to side against my clitoris. He kept saying, 'It's amazing . . . it's so smooth . . .' His eyes were really lit up, and because he was so excited, I started to get excited, too. I reached down with both hands and opened up my cunt lips for him. He rolled his cock around a little more, but then he positioned the head of it between my cunt lips and slowly pushed himself inside me.

"Do you know what the greatest thing was? For the first time I could really feel Brad's balls thumping against me, and it was so exciting. He couldn't get in deep enough. He fucked me like that for a while, but then I said, 'Roll over . . . lie on your back.' That was the first time that I had ever told him what to do in bed, but he didn't murmur. He just rolled onto his back, holding his cock up so that I could sit on it. It was dark red and shining with juice. I hunkered down over him, opening up my cunt lips with my fingers, and I looked down and watched as his cock slid into my totally hairless cunt. I saw down on it, right up to the balls, until it looked as if I *did* have pubic hair—his.

"Riding on top of him was beautiful. My breasts bounced, and Brad was able to hold them and squeeze them and lick my nipples. If I sat with my back straight his cock went so deep that it made my stomach feel weird. If I leaned forward, I could feel him pushing against my clitoris. I had never been so much in control before . . . and all because I'd shaved my cunt and turned him on so much.

"I rode him faster and faster. His hands gripped my ass and one of his fingertips poked into my asshole. I was panting now, and gripping him tight between my thighs, and he was pushing himself so hard and fast that I knew he was going to have to come. He suddenly shouted, and I felt his cock throb right inside my cunt.

"I leaned forward and we held each other tight, kissing each other like we hadn't kissed since we first met.

I felt Brad's cock soften and slowly slide out of me, and I could feel his sperm dripping out of me, too. I hadn't come, but it had been so exciting that I didn't really mind. But Brad said, 'Come on, baby. I haven't finished yet. You can't look this good and expect me to leave you alone.' He turned me over onto my back and opened my legs and started to kiss me and lick me, even though my cunt was filled to the brim with his own sperm.

"I lay back and I seriously thought that I was in heaven. Lying naked on a huge luxurious bed on a sunny Florida afternoon, with a naked, good-looking man licking my cunt as if he wanted to eat it. I had a wave of orgasm, and then another, and then another. I wanted him to stop but I didn't want him to stop.

"I thought it was all over, but he turned me around so that I was kneeling doggy fashion on the bed. He reached over and picked up a bottle of suntan oil from beside the bed. He poured some into the palm of his hand and then he smeared it between the cheeks of my ass, sliding his finger in and out of my asshole. Then he smeared it all over his cock, too, which looked even harder than it had been before. He didn't say a word, but he put the head of his cock up against my asshole, and he pushed it in . . . only a little way at first, only about an inch. I could feel my asshole gripping his cock, and I didn't know if I was going to be able to take him all in. But he pushed again, and then again, and this time I pushed, too. His cock went so deep into my ass that I couldn't help shivering. He reached around and started to caress my cunt, playing with my clitoris, stretching it and tugging it, and all the while his cock was so deep inside me. I felt as if I was having an orgasm and a huge movement both at the same time . . . like nothing I'd ever felt before.

"I started to shake and I couldn't stop shaking. Brad began to fuck me in the asshole in earnest now, in and out. I thought I couldn't take any more but it went on and on, until finally I felt sperm spraying all over the backs of my legs and the cheeks of my ass, and Brad collapsed onto the bed beside me.

"We made love every night that whole vacation . . . and most afternoons, too. Those two weeks really turned our relationship around. Do I think it'll last? Well . . . Brad's asked me to marry him, and I'm looking forward to a fall wedding. I'll tell you something, though. Underneath that white wedding dress, my cunt will be bare. Brad wouldn't have it any other way, and neither would I."

Of course Renata's relationship wasn't saved just by a shave. Although her relationship with Brad had started to fray at the edges, they still loved each other and they still had the will and the potential to enjoy all of the basic ingredients for a creative and exciting sex life. All they needed to do was to look at each other with fresh eyes. They needed to make a positive effort—yes, even an *exaggerated* effort to show that they still found each other sexually attractive.

Taking a vacation was an excellent idea. It's remarkable how many couples who think that their sexual relationship is growing stale find that a few days away can revive all of the romance and the sensuality that they thought they'd lost. On a vacation, your partner *has* to pay attention to you, and it's then that, like Renata, you can arouse his interest with a little sexual display, such as shaving.

Women who don't want to shave can still find a way to catch their partners' eyes. Sherri, a twenty-five-year-old dancer from Austin, Texas, wrote, "I tie little red silk ribbons in my pubic hair . . . my boyfriend loves the way it looks and he loves the way it *feels*, too. He says the sensation of all those little bows tickling him is too much!"

Nadine, a nineteen-year-old student from Detroit, Michigan, said, "I always have colored beads in my hair so I decided to try knotting colored beads into my pubic hair, too. My boyfriend thought it was so sexy that I've kept them in ever since."

Other women decorate their vulvas by piercing them with studs, rings, and chains. Stefanie, a twenty-eight-year-old artist from Sausalito, California, said, "I had my pussy lips pierced about five years ago with two gold rings that are joined together with a gold chain. The chain is connected with a small padlock and the only person who has the key is me. You wouldn't believe how much it turns my partner on to have to ask me for the key every time he wants sex. Or *beg* me, sometimes. He can be kneeling between my legs, holding his big hard cock in his hand, and he can't do anything until I let him in."

Charlene, a twenty-four-year-old jewelry store assistant from Dallas, Texas, has her ears, her nose, her tongue, and her eyebrows visibly pierced. "I also have rings in my nipples, a ring in my navel, and six rings in my cunt. Believe me, I have no trouble attracting men. They look at the rings in my nose and they raise an eyebrow. Then I nod toward my breasts, and give another nod further downward. You should see their faces! I'm not beautiful, by any stretch of the imagination, but they're panting for me!"

Piercing, I hardly need mention, should always be carried out by a qualified practitioner with new or sterilized needles. If you fancy the look but you don't relish the idea of actually being pierced, you can buy gold-plated clips that fasten onto your labia and that have two dangling gold chains with semiprecious stones mounted on them. You can buy clip-on nose jewelry and nipple chains, too.

A woman might draw her lover's attention to her pubic area with tattoos. Various designs include coiled serpents, hummingbirds, and even bees clustered around the vulva as if they're attracted to a woman's "honey pot." Rose petals are a favorite, too. Again, if you don't want to go to the extreme of actually being tattooed, you can buy washable tattoos that look just as good as the real thing.

Sandy, a twenty-five-year-old riding instructor from Denver, Colorado, said that she occasionally inserted a large fresh daisy in her anus as a way of making herself look more decorative before she made love—"Pink ones look gorgeous", and Georgina, a twenty-three-year-old research assistant from Washington, DC, said that her partner became "very excited" when she took him to bed with crimson ostrich feathers sticking out of her anus. "I took four plumes, tied them together, and then I bound up the ends with tape. I fitted a latex vibrator cover over them . . . one of those covers that's shaped like a man's cock . . . so when I put them in, *I* get a whole lot of pleasure out of it, too. Dan loves the way they tickle, and he says that they make me look totally decadent, you know, like something out of an old-time brothel."

Susan, nineteen, a student from Santa Cruz, California, said that her boyfriend loved it when she pushed the handle of a soft-bristled hairbrush into her anus, so that his scrotum was vigorously brushed during lovemaking.

You'll notice that all of these women made themselves a little bit more sexually exciting of their own initiative—not because their partners had asked them to. They were daring, they were sexually adventurous, and that's what made such an impression on the men in their lives. Don't wait until your partner says, "I'd love it if you wore a diamond stud in your cunt," or "How about sticking a flower into your asshole," because he never will. Either he'll be too reticent to suggest it, or else it won't even occur to him. The sexually irresistible woman is sexually *creative*—she's like Martha Stewart, always thinking of new ways to excite her man's attention.

Kelly, twenty-three, a law student from Los Angeles, California, gave her boyfriend a birthday that he'll never forget. "I invited him to my apartment for a birthday supper. When he arrived the whole place was in darkness . . . except for the bedroom. He came into the bedroom and there I was, waiting for him, completely naked except for my red high-heeled shoes. I was lying back on the bed with one big red candle up my cunt and another up my ass, both of them lighted, my legs wide apart, singing *Happy Birthday*. I'll never forget his face. And I'll never forget what happened after he blew out the candles!"

Not many women are as lighthearted about sex as Kelly, and that's a pity. Although most sexual relationships have serious overtones—love, loyalty, jealousy, possessiveness, domination, and submission—the most irresistible women are those who don't take sex too seriously. They are much more in control of their sex lives, and much more in control of their lovers.

In other words, if you spend your All-Day Self-Pleasuring Session trying to rid yourself of all of your hang-ups and inhibitions about sex, you will end up being in charge of your own body, and in complete control of your own sexuality.

Take a break now. Make yourself a cup of coffee or

pour yourself a soda or even indulge yourself in a midmorning glass of wine. Why not? There's nobody around to say that you can't. While you're drinking your coffee, allow your hand to stray between your legs and play with yourself. Enjoy yourself. Enjoy the feeling. Why not slip your vibrator up you, too, and slide it in and out? There are few things more erotic than pleasuring yourself in your normal day-to-day surroundings, in complete privacy.

After your break, it's time to think of dressing up. Maybe you never thought of buying erotic underwear before. Maybe you never considered that rubber or leather was quite "you." But it's surprising how many women—once they've taken the plunge and tried it—find sexy underwear and fetish clothing very arousing.

For her All-Day Self-Pleasuring Session, Nancy had bought herself a selection of bras and basques and panties from a mail-order company advertising in a woman's magazine. You'll remember that Nancy regarded herself as having something of a weight problem, so this was the first time that she had ever considered dressing in erotic underwear. "I just used to look at all those wispy panties and all those lacy bras and think that they could never be for me." But she was surprised to find that many of the garments she selected were extremely figure-enhancing. "For the first time ever I looked at myself in the mirror and thought that I looked really sexy."

Her favorite was a black latex bodysuit. "I wasn't at all sure about wearing rubber at first, but once I managed to get into it I changed my mind. That bodysuit flattened all the parts of me that I wanted to be flattened, but it left my breasts completely bare. I have *very* big breasts but this was the first time they'd looked really spectacular. Black rubber, white breasts, red nipples. It really was something. I wore thigh-length rubber boots, too, with four-inch heels. Just the thing for treading on a man's chest! But what I liked best about the bodysuit was that the crotch was open, which was very erotic. Most of the time it looked like it was closed, but then you could sit with your legs slightly apart and suddenly you would have a hairy pussy peeking out from the slit in the rubber. I think I'd defy *any* man to not find that a turn-on."

But she was also pleased by a black lace basque, which again left her breasts completely exposed, worn with black stockings and high heels. She was less sure about a selection of G-strings ("I just don't feel comfortable in them") but she liked several different high-waisted and high-cut panties and thongs, including a pair of open-fronted white lace briefs and a white leather pair that laced up at the sides.

So you don't have a cover girl face? So you don't have a Playmate figure? That doesn't mean that you can't look dramatically sexy—that you should never bother to dress in anything except "practical" clothes, or neglect your hair, or forget about your grooming. Because every single day that you go on believing that you'll never look sexy is one more day that you'll pass up the chance of attracting the kind of man you really want. No man is going to find you sexually attractive unless you *are* sexually attractive, unless you *feel* sexually attractive—and, as we've already seen, sexual attraction has very much less to do with looks than it has to do with radiating your sexual self-knowledge and your sexual self-confidence. Sexually self-confident women dress to make the best of their femininity. They style their hair to suit their faces. They always look smart and fresh, and carry themselves as if they're in charge of their lives. They have setbacks, for sure, because life is cruel and men are thoughtless and things seldom work out like they do in the movies. But think of all the famous, attractive women you know who are very much less than oil paintings. Bette Midler, Barbra Streisand, Oprah Winfrey, Karen Black . . . none of these women lost their sexual self-confidence because of their less-than-perfect looks.

Listen to what kind of women movie actor Jack Nicholson finds the most alluring: "I love the way women walk and move and smile. I just find it intoxicating. Watching a woman sitting in a café or walking down the street in a short skirt or an open blouse is one of the many minor thrills that women provide for men. And when you fall in love with a woman who turns you on that way, that's about as good as it gets."

Nancy never thought that she would dress in erotic underwear, but when she did, it made her feel as if she'd at last acknowledged what she really was: a very feminine, very highly sexed woman. "I suppressed my sexual feelings for so long because I never thought that I could attract a man. I took my mirror at face value and always thought that I was going to be fat and dowdy. I'll admit that I still haven't lost too much weight. I'm trying, but I don't find it very easy. But it's been a whole lot easier now that I know that I *can* be sexy, that there's more to me than my mirror image."

Nancy's right, of course. Your mirror shows you what you look like. It doesn't show you what you are. You should never make a judgment about yourself based solely on what you see in the mirror. Your reflection won't show you your warmth, your personality, your sexual aura.

You'll recall that Linda was aroused by the idea of making love to a much younger man. Her first instinct was to dress young. But young men are attracted to older women because of their sophistication and their maturity, and because they assume that an older woman will already know what to do when it comes to sex. For that reason, I suggested that Linda try to act her age. She was forty-two—what's wrong with being forty-two when you have smooth skin, silky hair, a good figure, and you *feel* like you're fifteen years younger?

Linda bought herself a selection of erotic underwear, but hers was all satin, lace, and silk. "It always gives me a good feeling, buying new underwear. But this was very special. I bought pinks and peaches, mostly. They were beautifully made but they were also very sexy. A quarter-cup bra that left my nipples exposed. A bra with holes for my nipples to poke through. A wonderful pair of panties—silk, with a lace edging, but no back on them at all, only a string of elastic. Open panties, a G-string made of embroidered Swiss lace, and a pair of crimson satin panties with a single circular hole at the back, so that a man could have anal intercourse with you and you wouldn't even have to take off your panties."

Linda said, "I may be forty-plus, but I still feel the same as I did when I was twenty-five, and I still have the same sexual urges. But of course I've been feeling less confident because I know, deep down, that I can't attract men the way I used to. Wearing really sexy underwear has done a lot to make me feel better. It's that hidden thing, isn't it? It's walking into an editorial meeting and knowing something that nobody else knows—neither the men nor the women. The men would probably cream their pants if they knew and the women would probably be scandalized. Underneath that severe chalkstripe skirt, I'm wearing nothing more than a tiny pair of lacy panties with two embroidered holes in them—one for pleasuring my cunt and the other for pleasuring my asshole. I have no pubic hair whatsoever, and a small tattoo of a bluebird just above my clitoris.

"It's *knowing* that, it's *knowing* that you're sexy, that gives you the power. You're not sexy because men tell you that you're sexy. You're sexy because you *are* sexy. It comes from inside of yourself."

Here's Beverley, a thirty-eight-year-old computer programmer from Sacramento, California. "Matt and I had been married for eleven years and I guess you could say that our sex life had settled into kind of a comfortable rut. We usually made love only once or twice a week, or sometimes when it was a special occasion, like we were on vacation or something or maybe it was my birthday. But I have to say that all the real fire had gone out of it. It didn't excite us the way it used to, when we couldn't keep our hands off each other.

"I wasn't desperately frustrated, but I was disappointed. I'd always had the idea that we would be having good, exciting sex right up until the time came for us to go to the sunset home, you know? I was talking with my best friend, Barbara, about sex, and Barbara was complaining that her husband, Michael, just wouldn't leave her alone. 'He wants it just about every night.' But then she said, 'I guess it's my own fault, really. I do like to tease him. But you have to keep a man's interest up, don't you—not to mention his cock.' It turned out that she almost always wore erotic underwear, and that she was always strutting around in it when it came to bedtime, and sometimes she would give him a full-blown striptease, with music and everything.

"It had never occurred to me that *I* could do anything like that to liven up our sex life. Wearing sexy underwear and stripping ... that was something that other women did, and I hadn't even been able to imagine what kind of women they were. When Barbara told me that *she* did it—and Barbara's the most respectable person you could ever hope to meet—well, I have to admit that it was some surprise.

"She lent me two of her erotic underwear catalogs. Some of the underwear was quite traditional—you know, basques and lacy panties. But some of it was quite far out, like crotchless catsuits and fishnet pantyhose that left your tushy bare. At first I felt very guilty and strange about the whole thing, but I have to say that the catalogs turned me on. The idea of really wearing underwear like this ... well, it was exciting, and in the end I thought, I'm a grown-up woman, I can do what I like, why not? I ordered two bras—one was a quarter-cup in black lace, and the other was white see-through nylon. The cups had vertical slits so that your nipples would poke through. I ordered a black lace crotchless catsuit, and three G-strings. I also ordered a black garter belt and black stockings.

"Barbara said it would probably be better not to try a full striptease on the first night. 'You don't want to give the poor guy heart failure.' She said I ought to act casual, just walk around in my new underwear as if it was the most natural thing in the world, as if I *always* wore underwear like that. 'Of course you'll be flaunting yourself,' she said. 'But he's going to have to make the first move. You won't make him feel like some useless joe in a striptease theater who can only sit there and watch.'

"On the first evening, when Matt came home I was wearing one of my simple black dresses, but underneath I was wearing my garter belt and stockings and my quarter-cup bra. I was nervous about what was going to happen, but I was very, very excited, too. My cunt was so wet that halfway through the evening my G-string was soaked, and I hadn't been *that* wet for a long, long time.

"Matt was pretty tired that night and usually there wouldn't have been much chance of him making love to me. When it came to bedtime he undressed first and sat on the bed in his pajamas watching TV. I went up to him, turned my back, and said, 'Could you unzip me?'—which he did, hardly looking. But then I drew my dress over my head and walked toward the bathroom, without turning around, and I heard him say 'Heyyy . . .'

"It was then that I turned around, so that he could see that although I was wearing a bra, my nipples were completely exposed. You should have seen his face! But I didn't give him the chance to say anything else . . . I just went into the bathroom and started to brush my hair in front of the mirror.

"Matt was into the bathroom before you could say 'Gypsy Rose Lee.' He came up behind me and put his arms around my waist and I could feel his cock rising up inside his pajamas. He said, 'These are new, right? Where did you get them? They're sensational!' He couldn't stop ogling me in the mirror, and his cock grew so stiff that it came out of his pants; I could feel it against my bottom. I tried to act cool, the way that Barbara had suggested. 'I just felt like something new, that's all . . . and Barbara lent me a couple of her catalogs.'

"Matt was amazed. '*Barbara* wears underwear like this?' he said. 'No wonder Michael always has a smile on his face!' He kissed my shoulders and then he raised his hands and touched my breasts so that my nipples pricked up. He kept on kissing me and kissing me and he couldn't get enough of me. It was like he wanted to eat me alive. He reached down between the cheeks of my bottom and tugged the elastic of my G-string to one side. Then he opened up my cunt with his fingers and pushed his cock right up me. He was so forceful it was almost like being raped, except that I wanted it, I really wanted it. I bent forward over the bathroom basin and opened my legs as wide as I could. Matt literally tore off his pajama pants, and then pulled off his top, so that he was completely naked. He wound his hands into my garter belt, and gripped me by the hips. He fucked me like he hadn't fucked me since we first met. I was so wet that every time he pushed himself into me there was a loud kissing noise. And I could actually *see* myself being fucked, in close-up, because it was right in front of the mirror. I could see my eyes sparkling and my breasts bouncing up and down in my quarter-cup bra.

"He started to fuck me faster and harder, and I knew that was a sign that he would be climaxing soon. So I did something else that Barbara had told me to do. I turned around, so that his cock came right out of my cunt. I think he was just about to protest, but I took hold of his cock with my left hand and held it real tight. I led him back into the bedroom and gently pushed him so that he was lying on his back. I sat astride him in my shiny black stockings and I rubbed his cock three or four times. Then I bent forward and took it in my mouth. I slowly sucked it and licked it and ran my tongue all the way down it, until it was glistening with my saliva. Then I held it in my hand and climbed on top of it, so that it slowly slid all the way up inside my cunt.

"Barbara had said, 'Make love to him in the way that's best for you—he'll enjoy it, whatever you do, but you'll be making sure that you enjoy it, too.' So I fucked him in a very slow and complicated rhythm, you know—using my cunt muscles to give him all kinds of squeezy feelings. He wanted to fuck me faster, but I was on top and I wouldn't let him. I wanted my own climax to build up first.

"I really let myself go that evening. I fantasized that I was a whore and that Matt was my customer. I fantasized that there were other men waiting outside the bedroom and that as soon as Matt was finished they would come in and fuck me, too. Before I knew it, I was gripping Matt's hips between my thighs and I was shaking and quaking in one of the most wonderful orgasms I'd ever had. Matt started to fuck me really fast now, ramming himself right into me, and the feeling was almost too much to bear. I had another orgasm, and then another, and then Matt let out this amazing shout and I could feel his cock pumping.

"We lay side by side for a long time afterward, just holding each other and kissing. Matt said, 'What happened to you, you suddenly started dressing so sexy?' and all I could say was, 'I was always sexy. I just dressed this way so's you'd notice.' "

Three nights later, Beverley tried her first striptease, dancing to a slow samba and gradually peeling off her new underwear piece by piece. We'll talk about striptease techniques later, but as Beverley said, "It worked like magic."

Many women are reticent about wearing erotic underwear because they think it makes them look cheap and obvious. "Only whores wear crotchless panties." But the truth is that it's one of the best ways of showing your man that you're still interested in arousing him sexually and that you yourself are still sexually arousing. It took only a garter belt and a pair of black stockings for Beverley's husband to be jolted back to the realization that he had married a very sexually attractive woman.

There's nothing whorish about dressing to excite the man you love—and, again, it's one of those things that gives you much more control over your love-making. You choose what you want to wear, and when and where you want to wear it. You choose whether you want to look like a courtesan or a maid or a slave or a dominant woman in black stockings and uniform.

Beverley felt so much in control of her lovemaking with Matt that she confidently used two delaying techniques to make sure that he didn't climax before she was satisfied. The first technique was to take his penis out of her and grip it very tight (we'll see more of this technique in just a moment). The second technique— surprisingly, perhaps—was to give him oral sex. Both of these techniques *look* highly stimulating, which is important if you don't want your man to feel frustrated or resentful. But for most men, the *look* of oral sex is much more arousing than the actual physical stimulation that it gives them. If you give your partner very gentle licks and laps with your tongue, with no manual stimulation, you'll slow up his climax rather than accelerate it. I'm not saying that he *won't* climax, but he won't climax as quickly as he might have with the full thrusting of intercourse.

You'll recall Ella, from our last chapter. Ella's problem was centered around "the stimulation gap"—the difference in time it usually takes for a man to ejaculate and a woman to experience a climax. Because Ella was so pretty and so sexually attractive, she found time and time again that her lovers would ejaculate long before she was ready to have an orgasm, a sequence of unsatisfactory sex acts that left her feeling "drained and frustrated. I felt used . . . like nobody cared about *me* anymore."

Ella didn't have to worry about arousing her lovers. Instead, she had to concern herself with two things: (a) how to slow down her lovers so that they didn't climax until she was ready for them; and (b) how to stimulate herself so that she could reach orgasm more quickly.

As far as slowing down her lovers was concerned, I recommended that in the early stages of lovemaking she should frequently change position—underneath, on top, sideways—so that she would constantly interrupt her lover's rhythm. She could also talk to him, telling him how much she liked him, and how glad she was that she had met him. Distracting, affectionate small talk, designed to take his mind off the job. She shouldn't, however, talk dirty, which might arouse him even more rapidly.

Another good way of delaying a man's climax is to use my own interpretation of the famous "squeeze" technique devised by veteran sex researchers Masters and Johnson in their treatment of premature ejaculation. Take his penis out of you and grip it very tight, right behind the head, with the ball of your thumb pressed hard against the hole. Keep on gripping it, as hard as you can, and at the same time pull down on the looser surface skin so that the head and shaft of his penis are being stretched. Keep on squeezing, while at the same time you gently play with yourself, right in front of him, making sure that he sees how you do it, and how much you like it. He won't see this as coitus interruptus . . . it'll all seem like part of your love play.

In effect, you're keeping him on "pause" while you catch up. When you do, you can guide his penis back into your vagina and resume your lovemaking as usual.

I used Ella's love of the great outdoors as a way of encouraging her to stimulate herself more quickly. One of her problems was that she lacked the ability to fantasize very strongly. Some women can create erotic fantasies in their mind that (combined with masturbation) will bring them to orgasm in the space of only a few minutes. But Ella didn't have that kind of a mind. She was a nurse, very analytical—trained to think of other people's welfare instead of her own.

Ella was lucky to have a small balcony at the back of her apartment where she couldn't be seen. She went outside completely naked and spent a sensual half hour massaging herself with perfumed oil, listening to music, and enjoying the late morning breeze on her bare body.

"It was out of this world," she said. "I lay back with my eyes closed and my legs open, and I could feel the wind caressing me. I slowly masturbated myself and I felt like I was in some kind of heaven."

CHAPTER SIX

The Pleasure's All Yours

One of the reasons that I recommend an All-Day Self-Pleasuring Session is because—when it comes to making love—it will help you focus on what turns you on the most. What stimulation, what location, what fantasies, what clothing, and what special aids, such as vibrators or erotic videos. When you make love, you will be able to think back on the ways in which you pleasured yourself during that All-Day Session, and you will know from experience how to intensify your pleasure. Some of the ways in which you aroused yourself in private may be too extreme for you to try with a man. For instance, you may have used a variety of phallic objects instead of a vibrator or a dildo—such as cucumbers, or carrots, or shampoo bottles, or jars of olives, or (in several cases) flashlights, switched on, so that they illuminate your vulva while you masturbate. You may not want to tell your lover all about your various penis substitutes, but you can think about them while you're making love, and your memory will increase the intensity of your experience. As one girl put it, "I kissed him while he was making love to me, and thought: I used to fuck myself with a big zucchini . . . now I've got a real live cock."

Over the years, I have received scores of letters from women asking if they have done anything wrong by masturbating with inanimate objects . . . anything from soft drink bottles to vacuum cleaner tubes. There is absolutely no harm in it at all—provided the object is clean, smooth, and you can accommodate it in your vagina or your anus without any pain and without any danger of it becoming irretrievably lost. The objects don't even have to be inanimate. Margie wrote to me from Darien, Connecticut, to tell me that her boyfriend had once pushed six or seven freshly shucked oysters into her vagina and eaten them out of her one by one. "There was a whole lot of slurping and sucking. It still turns me on every time I think about it . . . it was all so slithery."

Ella was excited by the idea of openly going naked, and showing herself off. Some women who feel a similar urge pleasure themselves by becoming naturists, or posing for men's magazines, or appearing in porno videos. It is perfectly normal for women to want to display themselves sexually. Sharon Stone crossed her legs in *Basic Instinct* to show Michael Douglas that she was wearing no panties. That was fiction. But Marilyn Monroe rarely wore panties, and famous British fashion designer Vivienne Westwood arrived at Buckingham Palace to collect an award from Queen Elizabeth II and twirled up her dress to display that she was knickerless. The flamenco dancer Carmen Miranda was frequently thrown up into the air by her partner to reveal what Kenneth Anger, the author of *Hollywood Babylon*, dryly called "natural ventilation."

I spent over ten years editing *Penthouse* and other sex magazines, and out of hundreds and hundreds of models, I never met one who didn't pose willingly and eagerly, and enjoy what she was doing. They were all sweet, attractive girls, with plenty of character, and I didn't meet one who felt that she was being exploited. Of course payment was a factor, but it wasn't a crucial factor. If a girl didn't want to pose in the nude, she wouldn't, regardless of how much you offered her. As one centerfold told me, "It's the one real hold that women have over men, isn't it? A man can spend all evening trying to impress you, but all you have to do is take off your clothes and you've got them eating out of the palm of your hand."

In Sweden I knew several girls who worked for live-sex clubs. Some of them would walk naked among the audience, encouraging men to push vibrators up inside their vaginas and their anuses. Others would make love on the stage, giving ostentatious demonstrations of oral sex. Hanna, twenty-four, a live-sex performer from Göteborg, Sweden, said, "It's so refreshing to show yourself off to people. After all, what are we? We are all the same. What is so terrible about a woman's vagina or a man's penis? We all have one or the other. We all make love. And if it pleases us to watch each other make love, why should we worry about that? Who does it hurt?"

I recommended to Ella that instead of erotic underwear she should wear no panties at all, even at work. She was aroused by the feeling of being naked under her skirt, especially when her boss (the dentist) and her patients didn't know. "Sometimes—when there was a good-looking man in the chair—I felt like saying, 'Do you realize that I'm not wearing any panties?' But I managed to resist the temptation. What turned her on the most, she said, was going to work in the morning after making love. "I was leaning over this real handsome guy and he was looking up at me with his mouth wide open—well, he had to, he was fitted with dental clamps—and I knew that he was really lusting after me, you know? And at the same time, *very slowly*, my boyfriend's sperm slid out of my cunt and started to creep down the inside of my thigh. I guess my eyes must have given me away, because the guy winked at me. And all the time he was having his crown fitted, he couldn't take his eyes off me, while my boyfriend's sperm was sliding down my leg and into my sock. For one mad moment I felt like lifting my skirt and showing him that I was naked underneath, and saying, 'Look! my boyfriend fucked me this morning and my cunt's filled up with sperm! You want to give me some more?" But that's just one of those mad ideas that go through your mind when you're really turned on, and I just kept on smiling and giving him mouthwash."

Ella said, "In another life, I guess I could have been a stripper. I love walking around naked, and one of my fantasies is arriving at the theater on a glittering opening night. Everybody is dressed in tuxedos and furs, but I'm completely nude."

Many women have similar fantasies. In *The Story of O*, the erotic classic by Pauline Réage, O is so subjugated by her lover that he takes her to a ball completely naked except for a bird's-head mask over her head and a leash around her neck. Her sex is shaved and pierced with a ring. "There was also a very young girl, bare-shouldered, wearing a tiny pearl choker, dressed in the kind of white dress that little girls wear when they go to their first ball, she wore gilded sandals and was with a boy who made her sit down next to O. The boy took her hand and forced her to caress O's breasts, and O quivered under the cool hand; and then he made her touch O's sex, and the hole through which the ring passed; the little girl obeyed in silence. It was not until daybreak that Sir Stephen and the Commander had O get up, led her to the center of the courtyard, detached her chain and took off her mask: and, laying her down upon a table, possessed her, now the one, now the other."

It was obvious that Ella would be highly aroused by daring acts of public nudity, so I suggested that the next time she met her boyfriend she should take him up in the elevator of the building in which she worked, lift up her dress, and show him that she was naked. Or take him out in the country someplace and spend the day, the both of them, completely undressed—"climbing, wading in streams, making love in the long grass." For Ella, sex was equated with personal freedom, both physical and emotional. Because of her very attractive looks, however, most of the men she dated quickly became very possessive and restrictive. They saw her as a status symbol, as a possession, rather than a person, and they didn't recognize that she had strong sexual needs of her own that weren't entirely centered around *them*.

I suggested that during her All-Day Self-Pleasuring Session she should concentrate on her *own* sexual identity, and make herself a shopping list of all the times she should have come out and told her partner exactly how she felt. You can do the same. All it takes is a pen and a pad and the readiness to face up to the truth. For instance:

1) How many times has he climaxed before you, leaving you aroused but unsatisfied, and you haven't said a word?

2) How often has he changed position just when you were beginning to get seriously aroused?

3) How often has he touched you too roughly/too gently/in the wrong place?

4) How often has he said nothing at all during sex, and made you feel as if you're nothing more than an inflatable doll?

5) How often has he put you in a position that has made it obvious that he wants you to give him oral sex—and that he would be very upset if you refused?

6) How often has he climaxed in your mouth without warning?

7) How often has he insisted that you make love when you didn't particularly want to?

8) How often has he penetrated your anus without your really wanting him to?

9) How often has he criticized your appearance or the things you say?

10) How often does he enter you before you're ready?

11) How often does he talk about *himself*, and what he wants, instead of you, and what you might want?

12) How often has he forgotten to tell you that he loves you? (That hurts, doesn't it?)

13) How often has he failed to introduce you to his friends and business colleagues as if he's really proud of you?

If, like Ella, you can answer "too often" to more than six of these questions, then it's about time you asked yourself (a) if you're dating the right man, or (b) whether you need to confront him with all of his failings, or (c) whether there's any hope of your being able to discreetly teach him how to become the lover you always wanted.

Your answer will have to be based on your own experience of your partner's character—and, of course, how much you love him and whether you're prepared to make the effort to change him. But far too many sexual relationships are desperately unfulfilling for women because the women won't speak out, or because they don't dare speak out, not wanting to incur their partner's anger or lose him.

If the man in your life isn't giving you the sexual satisfaction you deserve, there are plenty of ways in which you can gently suggest that he improve his lovemaking. We've already seen how you can shift your body while he's making love to you to indicate whether he's pressing too hard, or touching you in the wrong place. We've seen some techniques for delaying your partner's climax. But sometimes you really have to come out and say, "Please . . . don't do that," or "You're hurting me," or "Let's try something else."

Katie, a twenty-three-year-old fashion designer from Pittsburgh, Pennsylvania, said, "My boyfriend always climaxed before I did, leaving me *so* frustrated. So one night, after we'd made love, I took hold of his hand and put it between my legs, thinking that he'd get the hint and masturbate me. All he said was, 'Yes . . . I can feel it. I sure shot a whole load this time, didn't I?' In the end I plucked up enough courage to say, 'Diddle me, go on.' And he said, 'Why? Haven't you had enough?' He genuinely believed that when he was satisfied, I was automatically satisfied, too. But he did what I asked him, and after only four or five minutes he gave me one of those small, lovely orgasms that you sometimes have when you masturbate yourself. It turned him on so much that he got another hard-on, and he made love to me all over again, and *I* had another orgasm, too. I'd been so mad at him for leaving me feeling so frustrated. But until I told him, he honestly hadn't known what he was doing to me. Or rather what he *wasn't* doing to me."

Ella said, "I'm always frightened of deflating a man's ego." But if you really like a man and you want your relationship to flourish, there may come a time when you have to open up to him and tell him the truth. Don't be afraid. If your partner really likes you, too, he won't feel slighted—especially if you make a point of flattering him at the same time. Anna, twenty-eight, from Seattle, Washington, was not a great lover of anal intercourse, although her boyfriend attempted it two or three times a week. Eventually she told him that he would have to stop because his penis was so much bigger than other men's, and she was too small to take him in. "He wasn't upset at all. He glowed."

Coming out straight with a sexual criticism may give rise to some sulky or temperamental scenes. You know how sensitive men can be about their sexual prowess. But if you're clear rather than contemptuous, if you're affectionate rather than resentful, and if he really thinks a whole lot of you, then he'll be only too happy to change his ways . . . especially if he can see for himself how much more you're enjoying your lovemaking.

The *worst* thing you can do is to suffer in silence. Ariadne, thirty-three, a homemaker from Chicago, Illinois, said, "My husband was always so rough. He had sex with me as if he were fighting me. I would always have bruises inside my thighs and finger marks on my breasts and my back. He used to push his cock into my mouth and almost choke me. I don't know why I never said anything. In every other way he was the best husband that you could have asked for. He was generous and funny and everybody loved him. But I dreaded going to bed every night, and after five years I had to leave him. I know I should have spoken out but I was afraid of what would happen if I did."

Rhoda, twenty-six, who worked for a New York discotheque, had almost the opposite problem. "Men were always so timid with me. I like all kinds of sex. You know, bondage and cross-dressing and a little playful whipping. I met this gorgeous guy at the club and he came back to my apartment with me. I guess he was straighter than most of the guys I know, but he was so handsome he was almost unreal. We made love and he had a beautiful body. A dark cross of hair on his chest. A real washboard stomach. And such a cock—really long, with a wedged-shaped head.

"We saw each other four or five times, and every time it was the same—him on top, me underneath, and a cigarette afterward. I felt like I was in a 1960s movie. So the next time I fixed up four pairs of handcuffs on the bed, top and bottom, and said, 'Why don't you lock me up and have your wicked way with me?' He did it, but he didn't look happy about it, and his way wasn't wicked at all. He just did the same old thing—him on top, me underneath. Afterward he reached for the key and unlocked my right hand, but I said, 'What are you doing? Is that it? Aren't you going to fist-fuck me, or drop hot candle wax on my nipples, or push a vacuum cleaner hose up my ass? I mean, what kind of sadist *are* you?'

"I suppose I was being unfair. But he had no sense of adventure, you know? He had no sense of *play*. All sex is play, and I was only playing. He was scared of me, you know, and more than that he was scared of sex.

"He said, 'I'm sorry ... I have to go to the bathroom.' But I took hold of his cock in my one free hand and said, 'You don't ... you can use me.' At first he didn't even understand what I was saying. Like, how many men would pay money to piss on a pretty girl? I gripped his cock tight and I wouldn't let him go and after a while he started pissing ... only a little trickle at first, onto my breasts. Then his cock started growing hard again, and he really gushed out. I pointed his cock at my cunt so that he could piss onto my clitoris and between my lips. Then I sprayed my breasts again, waving it from side to side over my nipples, and last of all I opened my mouth and he pissed all over my tongue and my teeth. I didn't swallow very much. I took a big mouthful and sprayed it all out again, like a fountain.

"He was turned on. I knew that he was turned on. But he couldn't handle this kind of sex at all. To him, sex wasn't playfully pissing in your girlfriend's mouth. Sex was making love the ordinary way, in silence, and then sharing a Marlboro. I ask you, piss is sterile, so which is the least healthy?

"I never saw him again, which is a pity. He didn't need anybody like me. But the sad part about it is, whoever he settles down with, they're never going to know what sex *can* be like, if you stop being afraid of it."

You'll recall that Barbara was also aroused by the idea of sadomasochistic sex, but not so much for play. After a very unhappy marriage, she was looking for sexual comfort in being dominated. She no longer wished to take responsibility for any relationship, and I suspect that, in a way, she partly blamed herself for the breakdown of her marriage and was looking for punishment.

Barbara wasn't a real masochist in the sense that she could never be sexually aroused by anything except cruelty. But she had recurring fantasies about being raped and molested, and when she *did* make love she found herself wishing that her partner would dig his nails into her, or tie her up, or slap her, or anally rape her. "I even had a fantasy that two men kept me tied up to a bed and then masturbated all over me, into my face, into my hair, into my mouth, all over my breasts, and then they climbed on top of me and kissed me and raped me, both of them. I masturbated and then I was so disgusted with myself that I took a long, hot shower."

In reality it would be almost impossible for her to find a man who would be prepared to hurt her and humiliate her in bed and at the same time be trustworthy and reliable and friendly during the day. Such men exist only in sexual fantasies.

There was nothing intrinsically wrong with Barbara's masochistic daydreams. We all have erotic fantasies from time to time, and sometimes they can be very extreme. A very elegant thirty-four-year-old realtor's wife from Forth Worth, Texas, had read in one of my previous books about a woman's fantasies of having sex with a horse, and confided in me that one of her most secret fantasies involved her having intercourse with a stallion in front of all of her society friends. "Everybody has gathered in the stables. They're all in tuxedos and evening dress, but I'm nude . . . except for my pearls. I lie back on a bale of straw and the stallion stands over me. Its penis is enormous, bright red and actually steaming. I open my legs as wide as I can and my groom guides the stallion's penis toward my vagina. It's so huge that I can't possibly take all of it. But the stallion thrusts its haunches and everybody screams and applauds. There's such a strong smell of horse and sex. I look down and see this huge dark penis filling me up. It hurts but I want more of it. It feels so good that I don't care if it kills me. It shoves in and out, and it smells even stronger of sex and excitement. But then the stallion shudders and whinnies, and his sperm comes bursting out from between my legs, as thick as condensed milk. All of my friends scream. Some of the women faint. I kneel in the straw and suck the stallion's penis while it slowly ebbs away."

I've had letters from women who daydreamed about making love to six or seven men at once, or who want to have a naked man chained to a wall in their cellar so that they can whip him and abuse him. I had a letter from a woman who was worried because of her repeated fantasy—when highly aroused—of using the excrement of a famous movie star as a dildo. "After my orgasm, I feel so disgusted with myself."

But none of these women have any reason to feel anxious or disgusted. Creating sexual fantasies in your head is a normal part of arousing yourself. Everybody does it, to a greater or lesser extent. Understanding your fantasies will help you enormously to understand your sexual personality, and if you can accept them for what they are, instead of feeling guilty about them, you will be far more self-possessed and confident.

Writing down your fantasies can give you an extraordinarily clear profile of yourself ... apart from arousing you, too. When women write me about their sexual daydreams, I have no doubt that they find it exciting, just as men do when they write letters to sex magazines, or people of both sexes do when they write to advice columnists to explain their sexual problems—some of which are real, and many of which are nothing but fantasies. "I had a three-in-a-bed romp with my twin sister and my husband . . . now I feel a burning sense of shame . . . what shall I do?"

During your All-Day Self-Pleasuring Session, think of your own fantasies. Your own most extreme fantasies. The fantasies that you wouldn't tell *anybody* about, not even your very best friend. If you have a talent for writing, or you've been thinking about becoming a writer, why not write them down? It's surprising what a revelation it is when you actually take your wildest sexual fantasies out of the darkness at the back of your mind and put them onto paper, where you can look at them in daylight. Nobody else is going to read them, so don't hold back. Like Barbara, with her masochistic fantasies, admit for once those erotic things that you think about when you're sexually excited. It'll help you to understand yourself and what you need.

Be graphic and descriptive when you write. Try to explain to yourself why your fantasies excite you so much. Write them down with *feeling*. That way, you'll not only learn more about your sexual personality, you'll actually improve your writing abilities. Your All-Day Sexual Self-Pleasuring Session is about discovering *you*—not only your sexuality, but your complete personality.

Here's an excerpt from a long series of fantasies written by twenty-four-year-old Margarita, a newly married librarian from Phoenix, Arizona. "I'm very rich, and I own a huge house. It takes twenty or thirty servants to run it, and they're all men. Blonde surfer types, black men, Latin men. Some of them have muscles like bodybuilders and some of them are very lean and athletic. Some of them are very hairy and some have no body hair at all. They're all very handsome, and they're all naked, because I won't allow them to wear any clothes. At dinnertime I sit at the end of a long oak table with candlesticks on it. Four men bring me my food on golden plates. It's a gazpacho soup. I beckon one of the men to step close. I take hold of his long penis and dip it in the soup bowl. Then I take it out and suck it. I give it a long, languorous suck and run my tongue all around it. Then I beckon another man to come close and I dip his penis in the soup, too, and suck *him*. I taste the wine the same way, by having a big black man plunge his penis into my wineglass, and then take it out, dripping with wine, so that I can lick it. The men wait on me hand and foot, and carry me everywhere I want to go. They bathe me; they undress me. At bedtime they gather around my bed for the privilege of being asked to make love to me. I can lie back and have as many men as I wish, two in my mouth, one in my vagina, and one in my ass; and when they've finished I can have more."

All of the men that Margarita had known, including her husband, had been opinionated, intellectual, talkative types. "Kenneth is so *intense*, you know? Everything in life has to have a meaning or an explanation. Sometimes I feel like having sex with a man simply for the sake of having sex. I like romance but I don't *always* want romance. Sometimes I yearn for good old-fashioned lust."

Margarita was able to improve her sex life with her husband by using one of my most tried-and-tested techniques. Now and then she would greet him completely naked when he came home from work, and press her hand over his mouth as soon as he walked in the door. She would take off his coat and have his pants open before he had time to protest, and she would make love to him right then and there on the hallway carpet.

If you're better at drawing or painting, try sketching your fantasies. Again, do your best to make your sketches detailed and vivid. One girl, an amateur artist from Santa Fe, New Mexico, sent me an extraordinary self-portrait in which she was lying naked on a couch while being intimately examined by tall, handsome aliens with huge erect penises. Another talented amateur from Orlando, Florida, painted a watercolor in which she was a medieval princess being ravished by two knights. With drawing, your only limitation is your imagination, and a remarkable number of women have told me that putting their fantasies onto paper has been a tremendously liberating experience. One woman said, "It's like telling a secret that you've kept bottled up for the whole of your adult life."

Greta, a thirty-one-year-old advertising executive from New York, dark-haired and very pretty, told me, "It's better than analysis. When you talk to your analyst, she interprets what you're saying and tries to explain it back to you. But when you draw it for yourself, there it is, explained. When I drew my first series of fantasy drawings, they weren't especially good. I mean you wouldn't hang them in the Guggenheim. But they showed me for the first time that I had some quite strong bisexual tendencies . . . that I was attracted not only to men but to certain very beautiful women, too. I'd never been able to explain that to my analyst. I'd never really admitted it to myself. But there it was, on paper. Drawings of good-looking men with great big hard cocks, masturbating while they stood around all of these gorgeous blonde girls with long flowing hair and big breasts and their legs wide open."

Greta's self-discovery led her to form three "tentative" relationships with other women. "Only one of them involved actual going-to-bed sex. The other two were much more sisterly, although there was kissing and hair-caressing and one of the girls had such amazing breasts I couldn't stop touching them and playing with her nipples. The going-to-bed sex was very different from going to bed with a man. It was all so leisurely and gentle. There came a moment when my girlfriend was lying back on the bed with her thighs wide open and I was licking and kissing her cunt. I suddenly realized why men are so drawn to women. I suddenly saw what it was that makes a woman so irresistible. Her softness, her smoothness, her warmth. The way a woman kind of invites you into herself. That was the word. If a woman looks *inviting*, I think she can have any man she wants. And maybe any woman she wants, too."

To go back to Barbara and her sadomasochistic fantasies, I suggested that she find a way of expressing them on paper, either by writing or drawing. (Some women use cassette recorders and explain their fantasies out loud, and that can be very effective, too.) Barbara eventually both wrote and sketched some of her more extreme daydreams. One of her drawings shows her in a classic heavy bondage situation, her hair tied up to a hook on the ceiling, her arms tied behind her back, her mouth gagged, her waist cinched in by a lace-up corset. She is being whipped across the thighs and buttocks by two naked men with oversized erections.

The interesting feature of Barbara's drawings, though, was that there was almost always another man watching the proceedings. He looked like an older man, ordinarily dressed. When I asked her who it was, she said that she liked to fantasize about being watched while she was being punished or abused, but I personally thought that this older man had more significance than simply that of being a voyeur. He was more like a judge or a father figure, watching over her to protect her from too severe a punishment.

In any event, it was clear that what Barbara needed at this stage of her life was to attract a mature man with strength of character—a man who would be prepared to take charge of their relationship and make her feel wanted and protected. In other words, she needed to convalesce, emotionally and sexually, from the "black years" of being constantly criticized by her ex-husband for being "domineering,' while at the same time all of the responsibilities for taking care of the family had fallen on her shoulders.

In looking for a father figure, there was no need for her to worry too much about finding a man with whom she could settle down and have a long-term relationship. What she needed was a man who could help her to recover her pride and her sexual self-esteem—and she needed him as soon as possible. If she tried to find a second husband, she would not only be narrowing her options but making commitments for which she wasn't yet emotionally ready. Right now, she was feeling fragile and defenseless, but she had great inner resilience, and once she'd recovered her sexual confidence and stopped blaming herself for what had happened to her, she would be able to go looking for a man her own age—a man who was opinionated, sexually exciting, and who would appreciate her strength rather than blame her for it. A man, in fact, like her husband had been, in the days before their marriage had gone wrong.

In your sexual relationships with men, it's important never to lose sight of your own strength and your own identity. But it's equally important to recognize that there will be times when you feel the need for a man who is a protector and a good companion as well as a lover—and that many men respond in a very positive way if you make them feel that they can look after you. You may not really need all that much looking after, but then finding and attracting a man has always had a lot to do with playacting, and if you pretend that little you could do with great big him to take care of you, you'll be surprised how readily he responds.

Barbara began by making herself look younger and more vulnerable. She was a little too old for the Waif Look, but all the same she was very slim and boyish, and if she cut her hair short she looked at least five or six years younger. I suggested that she dress simply and demurely, and she didn't object to that at all, because she felt she needed simplicity and quietness in her life. I also suggested that she look at herself in the mirror and realize how attractive she was: slim, well-groomed, with very striking eyes.

Her ex-husband had constantly criticized her small breasts, and she was desperately self-conscious about them. "He kept saying that I wasn't a real woman, not like my friend Georgia, who's a 40D." She had thought of wearing inserts in her bra, but personally I think that inserts are as ludicrous as men wearing foam rubber muscles under their T-shirts. Small breasts are just as beautiful as large ones, and they give a woman the opportunity to go braless and dress very temptingly, in see-through dresses and blouses, and with one or two more shirt buttons undone. Jack Nicholson would certainly approve.

I also encouraged Barbara during her All-Day Self-Pleasuring Session to practice on herself some of the submissive sexual acts that she had fantasized about, so that she could see if she really did enjoy any of them—and, if she did, to learn how to do them safely.

Halfway through your day, you can have a light lunch—and, yes, you're allowed another glass of wine if you really feel like it. Afterwards, spend an hour or so doing something completely normal, like calling your friends or writing up a business report or tidying your closet, but do it nude or dressed in some of your new erotic underwear. The idea is for you to realize that even when you're undertaking the most mundane of daily chores, you're still sexy and attractive. Think about it next time you're cooking or cleaning up in front of your partner—*Underneath these jeans and this workaday shirt, I'm naked.*

Sheila, twenty-one, a veterinarian student from Los Angeles, California, took my advice from an earlier book and always spends Saturdays nude or seminude. "Jim looks forward to the weekend so much I keep telling him to stop wishing his life away. But I love it, too. It makes me feel like I'm really desirable, you know? I mean, when Saturdays come, Jim can't keep his hands off me, and Saturdays were never like that before. He always wanted to spend his time in the garage, tinkering with his car." Sheila has lots of wavy brunette hair and is very big-breasted. "Actually, Jim's preference is for small-breasted women. He loves what he calls 'teentsy tits.' But I guess he made an exception in my case. What he likes most of all is for me to go totally nude with just my high-heeled slippers on. He's always touching my breasts when I'm in the kitchen, or putting his arms around me, and I think he must have a hard-on for most of the day. A couple of weeks ago I was making pastry so my hands were all floury and I couldn't do anything to stop him. He came up behind me and squeezed my breasts, and then he rolled my nipples between his fingers. I told him to stop because he was turning me on and I couldn't have sex right in the middle of making pastry. But he slipped his hand between my legs and started to stroke my pussy. I was juicy already, so when he stuck his fingers up inside me I was really ready for him. He finger-fucked me for a while, going really deep. Then he spread my lips open wide. With his other hand he opened up his pants and took out his cock and pushed it right up me. His cock was so hot and hard and I wanted it so badly that I stuck out my tushy and waggled it around so that he could push it in even deeper.

"His fingers were all slippery with pussy juice. He used the juice to massage my nipples and he gave me a feeling like I've never had before, like my breasts were all hot and tingling. I think I could have had an orgasm just from having my nipples massaged like that. When his fingers got dry he slid them into my pussy again, right next to his cock, so that they were all juicy again, and he could massage my nipples some more. He fucked me harder and harder. My breasts were jumping up and down and of course I couldn't think of cooking anymore. I was clutching the pastry so tight that I made deep finger marks in it. I could feel Jim's cock growing larger and larger, the way it always does before he climaxes. I could feel every ridge of it, every vein of it. My pussy felt so sensitive, and I could even feel his pubic hair brushing against the cheeks of my bottom.

"Then suddenly he gripped my breasts really tight and pumped his come into me. I was so frustrated, because I was just about to come myself, and I hadn't quite made it! Jim took himself out of me, and turned me around. There was a long string of white sperm dangling from the end of his cock, and I took hold of his cock in my hand and massaged the sperm all over his balls, the same way that he'd massaged my nipples.

"'You came, like, two seconds too soon,' I told him. 'Can't you get this up again?' But I knew that he couldn't, not just yet. So I took the rolling pin off the table, and said, 'This looks about the same size as you. Come on . . . see if you can make me come.'

"We have a small couch in the kitchen, covered with cushions, and I lay back down on it with my legs wide apart and opened up my pussy with my fingers. His come was dribbling out of me, right between the cheeks of my bottom, and I could smell it, like such a sexy animal smell. Jim took the rolling pin and buried one of the handles in my pussy. It was still all floury, but that didn't matter because I was so juicy anyway and full of sperm. Jim pushed the rolling pin right up inside me and started to fuck me with it, and at the same time he bent his head down between my legs and licked my clitoris.

"The feeling was sensational . . . I thought I was going to go crazy. I reached down and pulled my pussy lips wide apart so that I could see Jim's tongue flicking around my clitoris, and the way he was sliding that rolling pin in and out of my hole. My hands were covered in flour and pastry, but I couldn't stop myself from stroking his hair and his ears and touching his face. I even pinched my clitoris between my finger and thumb so that he could just lick the tip of it. His cock was sticking out of his pants and it was half hard and growing harder, so I took hold of it and rubbed it while he was licking me.

"Then it was all too much. I had an orgasm, and I could feel my pussy muscles gripping the rolling pin.

Jim kept on licking and licking and I had another orgasm, and then another. I was still holding his cock and it was then that he just spurted out more sperm—two long jets of it that spattered onto my stomach and my pussy. It was amazing just to watch it shooting out like that. This time I caught hold of him and took his cock into my mouth and sucked him hard, and while I was sucking him he spurted out a little bit more, which went straight down my throat.

"I don't go completely nude every Saturday. Sometimes I'll wear a little fuzzy white angora sweater and nothing else except high heels. Sometimes I'll wear panties. It makes it more exciting if you think of something different every week. If I have my period I'll wear jeans, but I'll still go topless so that Jim can fondle my breasts, and we still make love, although I prefer to have anal sex at that time of the month."

You can spend the afternoon of your All-Day Self-Pleasuring Session doing exercises—both sexual and nonsexual—and training your body to accept and enjoy all kinds of different sexual variations. If you can keep up a reasonable standard of personal fitness, you'll find that your lovemaking benefits enormously. You'll have greater stamina, greater physical flexibility, and you'll be able to make love in so many more positions (standing up, for instance).

You don't have to train to Olympic standards in order to enjoy your lovemaking more, and you don't have to be a contortionist. During the course of my research, however, I came across Mara, a twenty-five-year-old former athlete from San Francisco, California, who was so supple that she could lift her legs behind her head, bend forward, and lick her own clitoris. I had come across a painting by the famous erotic artist Jean Paul Goude of a ballerina doing much the same thing, and a number of reasonably lithe men are able to suck their own penises, but this was the first time that I had encountered a woman who could actually give herself cunnilingus to the point of orgasm.

"I've been doing it ever since I was fifteen or sixteen. I used to double myself up in bed and lick my clitoris until I came. It's something of a strain these days, but if I'm feeling really frustrated I can still manage it. I can only touch my clitoris with the very tip of my tongue, though. I'd love to be able to suck it, and to push my tongue up my own cunt, but that's beyond the bounds of physical possibility. I still fantasize about it, though. I'd love to drink my own juice, right out of my cunt."

One of the very best sexual exercises is vaginal weight lifting. The Dacomed Corporation makes weighted cones of various sizes that you can slip into your vagina. Your pubococcygeus muscle (more simply known as your PC muscle) automatically contracts and holds the weight in place. With regular use, the weights give your PC muscle more strength and flexibility, and can noticeably improve your lovemaking and the quality of your orgasms. You can grip his penis more tightly, you can squeeze it and almost massage it during intercourse, and your climaxes can feel much more intense.

During your afternoon of self-pleasuring, you should try making love to yourself with a dildo or a vibrator. Insert the dildo into your vagina and see how far you can draw it in by using muscular contraction alone, and then how far you can push it out. Try to see how long you can walk around your apartment with a dildo inside you—gripping it only with your vaginal muscles. Then lie back and play with it for a while, pushing it in and out as your partner would when he's making love. Which angle feels better? Which speed feels better? When you're making love for real, you rarely have the time to think if *this* position is more exciting than *that* position, or whether your partner is far too fast or far too slow. Now you can take the time to learn about your own responses.

"I love it when a man's cock is very hard and curves upward," said Linda. "You only see that in younger men, which may be one of the reasons I'm attracted to younger men. But having a curving-up cock like that means that they rub against the front wall of your vagina when they're making love to you, and I just adore that sensation."

Nancy found that her pleasure was intensified if she kept the head of her dildo just between her vaginal lips, teasing and taunting herself before allowing herself the pleasure of full, deep penetration. "That excites me . . . the idea of a man with a huge cock who will only give you just the head of it, and won't push it completely in, not until you're screaming for it, almost, and then he does, and you feel this gorgeous big thing forcing its way right up inside you."

Delaying full penetration can be a very exciting technique, and greatly intensifies both your passion and his. You may find that some men deliberately delay as a way of teasing and tantalizing you, but not many. A man's strongest urge is to push his penis in as quickly and as deeply as possible, and you won't find many men with the sexual skill to hold themselves back.

However, you can delay penetration yourself either by gripping his penis or by cupping your hands on either side of your vulva—so that when he first enters you, he is unable to go in all the way. With this technique, you will be in control of your own stimulation, and his, too—because it will be up to *you* to decide when to allow the entire length of his penis to enter your vagina.

You can also control how deeply his penis goes into you while you're in the middle of making love, especially if you've been toning your vaginal muscles.

You on Top: The best position for exercising control is when you're sitting on top of him during intercourse. If you practice this with your vibrator, you'll soon realize that when you lean forward his penis is unable to enter you so deeply, but that when you sit up straight it will go into you so deeply that it may even touch your cervix (the neck of your womb). You can also lift yourself up so that in order for him to penetrate you to the full length of his penis, he will have to thrust his hips higher and higher. When he's having to lift his buttocks off the bed to reach you, you will find that his penis darts in and out of you with a highly stimulating "flipping" motion. Keep on lifting yourself up until the head of his penis is barely penetrating your vaginal lips, and see how long you can hold yourself in that position before you sink back down again, burying his penis deep into your vagina.

You Underneath: If you are making love in the conventional man-on-top position, you can still have a considerable amount of control over how deeply your partner penetrates you. When you're lying flat, with your legs straight, it's difficult for a man to penetrate you very deeply—as you will be able to see if you practice with a dildo. This, of course, is why many women like to make love with a cushion or a pillow under their hips: to raise the angle of their vagina and to make it more accessible to their partner's thrusting. If you want to delay deep penetration, keep your knees lowered, your bottom flat against the bed, and bring your legs in closer together. As you become more aroused, all you have to do is lift your knees, lift your bottom, and open your thighs wider.

Side by Side: If you are making love side by side, either in the "spoons" position or with you lying on your side and him facing you on his side, it takes only a slight turn of your hips to increase or reduce the depth of his penetration. In the "spoons" position, you can retract your bottom if you don't want him to enter you so deeply, or push it toward him if you want him to go in further. Don't be afraid of using your hands in any of these situations. He won't mind at all if you hold his penis during intercourse, even if you're preventing him from penetrating you more than two or three inches.

Doggy Fashion: If you're kneeling on all fours and your partner is penetrating you from behind, you can control the depth of his thrusting by raising your head and arching your back, while at the same time clenching those well-exercised vaginal muscles of yours. If you want him to go in deeper, lower yourself down onto your elbows and lower your head. Lift your bottom so that he can plunge into you as deeply as possible.

Have your own private orgy with your dildo or vibrator. Feel all the best positions, and see if you can discover which positions make it easier for you or your partner to stimulate your clitoris during intercourse. It's not so easy when you're sitting on top of him, unless you've lifted yourself up a few inches, although it's a great deal easier when he's on top of you. He will be able to reach around and massage your clitoris while you're making love doggy fashion—but you'll find it difficult without losing your balance and toppling over. The ideal position for clitoral stimulation during intercourse is for you to be lying on your back with your knees raised and your partner to be entering you from one side. Then either of you can touch and play with your clitoris during lovemaking, and your partner will also find it easy to caress your vaginal lips or maybe even slide one or two fingers into your vagina alongside his penis. He will also be able to penetrate your anus with his finger or fingers and stroke his own penis through the thin wall that separates your vagina from your rectum.

Up until your All-Day Pleasuring Session, you may have thought about anal sex but never had the confidence to try it. Some women are very matter-of-fact about it and enjoy it regularly, particularly during that time of the month when vaginal intercourse can be a little messy. Other women dislike the whole idea of it—and if you're one of those, it doesn't matter at all. There are plenty of other sexy things you can do in bed, and you should never feel obliged to take part in any sexual act just because your partner wants to. It's your body, and if you don't want your lover's penis in your anus, then the decision is entirely yours.

Many women who *do* enjoy it find it a way of reaffirming their affection for their partners—almost like losing their virginity all over again. Cindy, twenty-four, an optician's assistant from Austin, Texas, said, "The night I let Ray make love to my asshole, that was the night when I knew that I was really his and he was really mine. We'd been married for a year and a half and our sex life was great, so there wasn't any need for us to try out anything kinky. I used to suck his cock almost every other day and he was always waking me up in the morning by licking my cunt. That particular night he came home with a huge bunch of flowers for no reason at all. We didn't do anything special . . . just had a couple of steaks and some salad for supper and watched some TV. But I couldn't take my eyes off him, I loved him so much. Well, I still do!

"We went to bed and started kissing and snuggling up together. Ray knelt over me and I took hold of his cock and kissed it. Then I took a condom out of the dish beside the bed, and rolled it onto his cock. I remember it was a bright blue condom, so his cock looked really amazing! I lay back and opened up my legs, and he pushed his bright blue cock into my bright pink cunt. He fucked me very slowly . . . that's one of the things he's learned about me, since we've been married. I always like to start off making love very, very slowly. When we first dated, he used to make love like a jackrabbit and I nearly didn't marry him because of that.

"In the end I slowed him down by taking hold of his balls while he was making love to me so that every time he thrust himself into me too quick and too hard, I tugged at his sack. Not too hard—I didn't want to hurt him—but just hard enough so that he would get the message.

"Anyhow, he made love to me beautifully. I just lay back with a dreamy smile on my face while he pushed his cock in and out of me. I lifted my legs higher and higher, and then I put them over his shoulders. I reached down with my fingers and opened my cunt even wider so that he could go deeper than ever. I wanted him to fill me up completely. I wanted to be stuffed full of solid cock.

"He climaxed. I was *nearly* there, but not quite. He lay down beside me and put his hand between my legs so that he could masturbate me, and I took off his condom and started to play with his cock. I love his cock when it's all soft and slippery like that. I massaged sperm all over his balls and his cock began to stiffen again, just a little. He was rubbing me quite fast now, and I could feel that it wasn't going to take me long before I had a climax. He slipped one hand under my bottom and started to finger my cunt and my asshole. His fingertip kept going around and around my anus and I pushed my muscles so that he could feel it opening up. He slid his finger inside, only an inch or two to begin with, but then he went deeper and deeper.

"I said, 'How about giving me something bigger than that?' He said, 'What?' and I said, 'How about your cock instead?' I had my hand on his cock when I said that, and you should have felt it. One second it was half-hard and rubbery. The next second it grew and grew until I thought it was going to burst. I reached over to the nightstand and took a tube of K-Y out of the drawer. Ray was so worked up that he was kissing me and rubbing my whole cunt with his fingers, which was absolutely fantastic. I squeezed out a handful of K-Y. It felt really cold and shivery! I smeared it all over the top of Ray's cock, and all around my asshole, too.

"Ray pressed the head of his cock between the cheeks of my ass, right up against my anus. At first my muscles were too tight to let him in, but then I pushed against his cock and the head of it slowly sank into my ass. The feeling was amazing. I couldn't resist reaching down and feeling all around my asshole, with his cock half-buried in it. It was stretched open so wide, but it didn't hurt at all. Ray said, 'Baby, you have the most beautiful ass in the whole wide world,' and he pushed his cock in another couple of inches. My muscles started to spasm, as if I wanted to squeeze him back out again. But he put his arms around me and kept us tight together. Then he pushed himself in again, and again, and I felt his pubic hair up against the cheeks of my ass. I reached down again and his cock was right inside my asshole, right up to his balls.

"Ray was great. He fucked me very slowly and gently, and whenever I tightened up he stopped. At first I couldn't stop my muscles from squeezing him, but after a while I began to relax, and he could fuck me properly, just like fucking my cunt. I turned over onto my side and sat in his lap, and pushed against him so that my asshole was wide open. His cock was so hard and so big—it felt like he was fucking me all the way up to my heart. It took him a long time to climax, too, because he'd just climaxed before, but when he did I climaxed, too, and that was the first time that the two of us had come together for a long, long time.

"That was a great night. I felt like we'd gotten so much closer together. It was a few weeks before we tried anal intercourse again, but when we did I was ready for it and I was able to open up my asshole and let him slide right into me, right up to the balls, without any pain and without any pushing. Now I don't know which I like the most: taking his cock in my cunt or taking his cock in my asshole. The other night he was fucking my asshole when he reached under the pillow and took out this big vibrator he'd bought, just like a man's cock, only bigger, and it never went soft! He opened up my cunt lips with his fingers and pushed it up me. I didn't know if I liked it at first. I felt like I was being *used*, do you know what I mean? I felt like Ray was treating me like a sex object. But then he switched on the vibrator and there was this deep, deep buzzing inside of me. It made my whole stomach quiver, and it made Ray's cock quiver, right inside my asshole, and before I knew it I was having a climax, and then another, and then another. I couldn't stop.

"Sometimes we do it the other way around, and he puts his cock in my cunt and the vibrator up my ass. I don't mind. It turns me on and it turns Ray on and we have the most satisfying sex life you could imagine."

Cindy showed that offering anal intercourse to your partner can be a way of showing that you have very special feelings for him. With a little perseverance, anal intercourse can be just as pleasurable as vaginal intercourse, and offers you a whole range of exciting variations.

Incidentally, Cindy's method of slowing down Ray's sexual thrusting by clutching his scrotum was a very interesting and effective technique. Another way of slowing down your partner's sexual speed is to reach around to his anus, stroke it, and then insert your middle finger. Slide your finger in and out of his anus at the speed that you want him to make love to you. If you want him to slow down, do it slowly. If you want him to do it more quickly, then thrust your finger in faster and deeper. Hurt him a little if you like. Slowly scratching his buttock cheeks close to his anus will slow him down, as will digging your fingernails into the skin of his scrotum.

Jayne, twenty-three, a supermarket manager from St. Cloud, Florida, said that she could always control the pace of her boyfriend's lovemaking by biting his nipples. "He loves it and he hates it, both. But it always stops him dead in his tracks."

There is always a strong element of domination and submission in anal intercourse, and the sexually irresistible woman knows how to use both in order to make herself much more arousing than any other woman her partner has ever met.

In his book on anal eroticism, the German author Helmut H. Lundberg quotes thirty-four-year-old Ingedore, who said, "I like it best when my husband plays 'smack bottoms' with me. What's that? It's our name for a favorite kind of foreplay in which we alternately slap the other's naked behind with gentle to light blows. Usually we already have vaginal coitus behind us when we begin the bottom slapping. After a short while my husband gets a second erection and flames seem to flare up in my pelvis. Soon I stretch my behind, which in any case he finds beautiful and attractive, invitingly toward him. After he has carefully inserted his penis anally, I usually determine the depth and the tempo of penetration. My husband is very careful and considerate to me. But I often urge him to get to work on my buttocks with the flat of his hand once he has got inside me. This often gives me an ecstatic orgasm which vibrates to the tips of my toes."

But many women don't realize that a man's anus is just as sensitive as a woman's, and that men can derive an enormous amount of erotic pleasure from having their anuses kissed or licked (anilingus, as it's known in the business) and from having a finger inserted into their anus during masturbation or oral sex. It's actually possible for a man to reach a climax by sticking his finger into his anus—a technique that was developed to a fine art by the inhabitants of the ancient Greek city of Syphnos, if classical illustrations are anything to go by. In fact the word "syphnosize" was coined to describe anal masturbation.

Lorna, twenty-eight, a music teacher from Louisville, Kentucky, discovered that if her partner's erection was flagging during intercourse, she could stiffen him up by inserting one or two fingers into his anus. "I guess men aren't used to the idea of somebody penetrating *them*, instead of the other way around. But it works ninety percent of the time. It also works if you're not quite satisfied and you want to make sure that your man has a second hard-on as soon as possible."

Emma, twenty-five, a very tall and pretty fashion model from Los Angeles, California, said that she had bought a strap-on dildo for the express purpose of penetrating her lover from the rear. "I was given the tip by a friend of mine, Jody, who works for a TV company. She was having an affair with her boss, who's very good-looking and very charming if you meet him socially, but he behaves like Attila the Hun when he's at work. I mean he probably has to, to keep the business profitable—but at the end of the day he's so stressed out that he needs somebody to calm him down, to make him feel good. He didn't make love to Jody for weeks, so in the end she decided that she was going to make love to *him*. She went to a sex store and bought one of these strap-on cocks. I mean what surprised her so much was that the store told her that most of them aren't bought by lesbians, to screw each other. In fact, hardly any. They're mostly bought by women who want to fuck their husbands and their boyfriends up the ass. And the men love it! That's what the woman in the store told her. And when she tried it on her boss, she said they had the most fantastic night of sex *ever*. They were at it all night . . . he fucking her and then she fucking him. And that was why I decided to buy one of my own.

"My boyfriend, Steve, is a very successful photographer, but that means he has to work all kinds of impossible hours, so like Jody's boss he's always too tired or too stressed to make love to me properly. I mean I love him for his personality as well as his body. Sex isn't everything, but sex is still pretty damned important.

"I bought the dildo mail-order and I didn't dare to

use it until about a week after it arrived. I could just imagine myself walking into the bedroom with a huge pink plastic boner and Steve falling over laughing. But one night he came home at two-thirty and I hadn't seen him for forty-eight hours and I was very excited because I'd just finished modeling this really sensational collection and I was *bursting* with adrenaline and I really wanted sex and what happened? He undressed and crashed out on the bed and fell asleep.

"So that was when I took off all of my clothes and strapped on this dildo. It felt really weird, having a cock sticking out in front of me, but it was kind of a turn-on, too. It bounced up and down when I walked, almost like a real cock. The only trouble was, it didn't have any feeling, you know? I didn't have any K-Y so I greased it up with hair gel. It was very big, bigger than a real cock, with bulging veins and everything. It even had balls.

"Steve was lying facedown, stark naked, fast asleep. I climbed on the bed and knelt between his legs. I opened up the cheeks of his ass and smothered his asshole with hair gel. Then I held on to the dildo and tried to push it into him.

"I couldn't believe how easy it was. There was a moment's tightness, right at the beginning, but then I leaned forward and there was a sticky kissing noise and the dildo went right up his ass. I don't know whether men find it easier to take things up their ass than women, but Steve took it, all of it, and at the same time his own cock uncurled itself and started to grow.

"I started to fuck him the same way that he would have fucked me. I dug my nails into his shoulders and I fucked his asshole until it was red. I put my hand underneath his stomach and found his cock and it was totally stiff, and it was pouring out slippery juice. I fucked his ass harder and rubbed his cock and then he shuddered like an earthquake and he climaxed—loads and loads of sperm, more than I'd ever seen him shoot out before, all over my hand, all over his stomach, all over the sheets.

"I carefully took the dildo out of his asshole, which was still sore and wide open. Then I bent down and I sucked his cock and licked the sperm from his hairy stomach and sucked it out of his pubic hair. I even licked it off the sheets, and then stuck my tongue out so that he could see it on my tongue. I think he thought he'd died and gone to heaven. He said, 'I never thought a woman could ever do that to a man. I wouldn't have believed it.'"

Women are learning at last that sexual assertiveness brings them the kind of relationships they want, and makes them irresistible to men. We're not talking about sexual *aggression*. We're simply saying that if you're unattached, and you go on waiting for men to initiate an intimate relationship, then unless you're very lucky, you may have a very long wait. Similarly, if you rely entirely on your partner to keep your sex life effervescent, your sex life may continue to be very flat.

Men need coaxing. They need encouraging. They need educating. Even the studs need to be taught how and when and where. Let's look now at how to finish off your All-Day Pleasuring Session, and how to use what you've learned to give your man the biggest shake-up since the San Francisco earthquake.

CHAPTER SEVEN

How to Give Him the Sex He Never Knew He Wanted

Every man has sexual fantasies, some of which can be quite straightforward, like a desire for oral sex, and some of which may be very extreme, like wanting to be whipped, or to wear women's underwear, or to crawl around the bedroom wearing a dog leash.

What makes a woman sexually attractive is knowing what those fantasies are and how to make them come to life. What makes a woman sexually *irresistible* is not only making those fantasies come to life, but giving her man new and unusual pleasures of which he never even dreamed.

Toward the end of your All-Day Self-Pleasuring Session, you should be thinking about all of those sexual acts that you'd really like to try, as well as those sexual acts that you're not totally sure about, but that you wouldn't mind experimenting with. This is the time when you can lie back and let your imagination really run wild, while gradually pleasuring yourself toward a final orgasm. This is the time for you to try to forget about all of your preconceptions and your inhibitions and allow yourself to think about some of those sexual acts that might have intrigued you or fascinated you or even shocked you.

There is no question that the single sexual act that men fantasize about the most is oral sex. Almost every sex magazine and video features pictures of girls sucking men's penises—sometimes two or three at once. Oral sex is particularly exciting to men because they are highly susceptible to visual stimulation and when you have your partner's penis in your mouth he can clearly see every suck and lick. Let's make no bones about it, oral sex has a strong element of subjugation in it—the woman showing her adoration of the man by taking his erect member between her lips—but this is a sexual response that we shouldn't get too political about. The plain fact is that when a woman is giving her lover oral sex, she is completely in charge of the intensity of his sexual stimulation and whether he climaxes or not and how quickly. So much for subjugation.

As we have already seen, you can use oral sex to control a man's sexual timing to quite a fine degree. If he's slow to raise an erection you can speed him up by sucking his glans (the head of his penis) and by vigorously rubbing the shaft with your hand. If you're having vaginal intercourse, and it feels as if he's approaching his climax too quickly, you can take out his penis and give it a long, slow suck to delay him without frustrating him. You can use oral sex to arouse him to a second erection if he didn't satisfy you the first time (or even if he did, and you simply feel like some more).

You can use oral sex as a substitute for vaginal sex if you're having your period or if you don't feel in the mood for penetrative sex.

Many women have written me to say that they're

hesitant to give their partners oral sex "because I don't really know how to do it." They're worried that they won't stimulate their partners enough, or that they'll hurt them, or that they'll look clumsy and amateurish.

You can give oral sex in any way you like, provided you remember that it's the glans—the head—that contains most of the hypersensitive nerve endings that will give your partner the most pleasure. Although oral sex is commonly referred to as "cocksucking," it's a combination of all kinds of stimuli—sucking, licking, and what you might call "lip fucking," when you use your lips and your mouth in the same way that you would use your vagina. The head of your partner's penis is not as sensitive to oral stimulation as your clitoris, which is why you will often find that he needs some manual masturbation of his shaft to bring him to a climax.

You can also insert your finger into your lover's anus while you give him oral sex, which will greatly intensify his feeling. Helmut H. Lundberg quotes thirty-nine-year-old Harald, who said, "It happened that during an hour of lovemaking my pretty-well-exhausted penis stood up again when my wife put her finger up my anus. Since then we have often indulged in cunnilingus or fellatio with the finger pushed up the rectum. My wife has acquired an almost unbelievable skill in satisfying me with mouth and tongue while she has her finger stuck up my rear. Meanwhile I have learned to repay her once we have got into the right position."

Oral sex is also known as a "blow job," but the one thing you should never do is blow into the hole in the end of your partner's penis. There is a very remote chance that you could cause physical damage or even give him an air embolism in his bloodstream, with fatal consequences. For the same reason he should never blow into your urethra or your vagina. Also, never insert any object into your partner's penis, apart from the tip of your tongue. Favorite urethral stimuli include the insertion of lubricated cotton swabs, ballpoint pen refills, or even plastic cocktail stirrers, but these can cause very painful tissue damage and a nasty infection. (And how are you going to explain *that* to your doctor?)

When you give your partner oral sex, the most important thing of all is to *relish* it. Too many women give their partners a quick, polite suck because they feel their partners expect it, and then insist on having vaginal intercourse. They don't realize how much pleasure and stimulation *they* could get out of it, if they took their time, and how much control it could give them over the pace and the intensity of their lovemaking. You couldn't enjoy a good meal if you gulped it down in a rush, so why not think of oral sex as a good meal, full of flavors and textures—something you want to savor.

Here's Gillian, twenty-one, who works for a video rental store in Dallas, Texas: "The first time I ever found out about oral sex was when I was sixteen years old. I was staying at home because I had a cold. My parents went out shopping and left me in the house alone. I was kind of dozing all afternoon, but around three o'clock I heard the front door open and I thought it was my parents. It was then that I heard the voice of my older brother, John, who was nineteen at the time. I heard a girl's voice, too. They went into the kitchen and I could hear them talking and opening the icebox. Then they went upstairs to my brother's bedroom. They obviously didn't realize that I was home. I heard them laughing and fooling around and then there was silence.

"I climbed out of bed and went to my brother's room. The door was half open so I could see through the crack. My brother was lying on his back on the bed wearing nothing but his T-shirt. His girlfriend was kneeling between his legs. I can remember her name— Jo-Anne. She was one of the prettiest girlfriends that John ever had. She was totally naked, except for her socks and her sneakers. She had heaps of blonde curls and a terrific figure—really big, round breasts and a waist like an hourglass and a big, round, suntanned bottom. She was sucking and licking my brother's cock, and she was doing it with such *gusto*, you know? Like her tongue was running all the way up from his balls to the top of his cock, and then she was swirling her tongue around and sucking it and even *chewing* it. She sank her front teeth right into the hole in his cock. Then she rubbed his cock all around her nose and her cheeks, kissing it and biting it. John was going crazy. His hands were gripping the comforter and he kept saying, 'Baby, oh baby, oh baby,' over and over again.

"Jo-Anne ran her tongue all the way down his cock and then she took one of his balls into her mouth. Remember that I hadn't seen my brother naked since he was about ten years old, and here he was with a huge purple-headed cock and this girl was sucking it and licking it and sinking her teeth into it. It was kind of like forbidden, you know; but being forbidden made it all the more exciting, and there was no question that John was enjoying it.

"Jo-Anne started to rub his cock up and down with her hand and lick it all around with her tongue. John went red in the face and said something like 'No— stop!' and held Jo-Anne's head. But she went on rubbing him and licking him and all of a sudden he was spraying sperm all over her face and into her mouth. He sprayed again and again, and some of it went into her hair and some of it went right over her shoulder and down her back. We'd been told about sperm in biology lessons but I'd never seen it before, not for real, and not shooting out of my own brother's cock. And what I couldn't get over was the way in which Jo-Anne licked it all up, and smacked her lips, like sperm was the most delicious thing she'd ever tasted.

"She went further up the bed and kissed him. She had her hand on his cock and she was still playing with it. She had sperm running down her back and sliding in between the cheeks of her bottom. I was *very* turned on. In fact I tippytoed back to bed and I masturbated. Like, I was at an age when the idea of sucking a boy's cock had always seemed like a pretty disgusting thing to do. But here was a girl who had not only done it, but really looked like she loved it. I'll tell you, that Jo-Anne made a big impression on me, so far as sex was concerned.

"I had my first serious boyfriend about a year later. Theo was really cool. He was very thin and very handsome and he wrote songs for this college band that he was in. He had brown curly hair that went right down to his shoulders. We dated a couple of times but he never came on strong. It was only when we went to a party one night that we actually got together and had sex. It was a huge party, in somebody's house. There was a lot of heavy music and drink and dope, but everybody was in a great mood and nobody was irresponsible, you know what I mean? We didn't have any jealousy or fighting or people going crazy, like you do sometimes.

"I guess it was about three in the morning and the

living room was practically dark. There were a whole lot of couples everywhere, kissing and cuddling each other. There was some really soulful rock playing from the other room. Theo held me and kissed me and we really started to get it on. He slid his hand inside my T-shirt and lifted up my bra so that he could play with my nipples. I could feel his cock inside of his jeans . . . it was huge, you know, like an iron bar or something. I tugged down his zipper and reached inside. I'd never done that before. I mean I'd felt guys' cocks inside of their jeans but I'd never had the nerve to open them up. I tugged his shorts out of the way and pulled his cock right out of his jeans. It was so big and hard that I couldn't believe it . . . and the smell of it, you know, it smelled like men's piss and men's sex, like an animal smell, and that really turned me on.

"I guess I was thinking of Jo-Anne sucking John's cock, because I put my head down and I took Theo's big fat cock right in my mouth and licked it all around. It tasted kind of bitter but that was what I wanted. I wanted the real taste of real cock. I started to suck him and lick him and rub his cock with my hand, the same way that Jo-Anne had rubbed my brother. Then I un-buckled his belt and pulled his jeans and his shorts right down to his knees, so that I could lick him and suck him all the way down to his balls.

"Theo couldn't believe it. He was moaning and groaning and I didn't know whether he was enjoying it or not, but when I lifted my head up he thrust his hand into my hair and pushed my head down again and said, 'Please, Gilly, please don't stop.'

"Somebody must have seen what I was doing, because it was then that they switched all the lights on, and there I was, right at the end of the couch, kneeling between Theo's legs and sucking his cock. I guess there must have been twenty or thirty people in that room, and they all let out this huge great roar, and started clapping. I could have died of embarrassment. Well, I *could* have died of embarrassment, but I didn't. I thought to myself: you want a show, I'll give you a show. You want to see how good it can be, to suck a man's cock? I'll show you.

"Theo started to go soft, but I looked up at him and said, 'No . . . let's show them,' and I took his cock back in my mouth and started to give him this long, strong, systematic sucking. He lay back on the cushions and closed his eyes. I guess he was trying to blot out the reality that there were thirty people watching his cock going in and out of my mouth. But it didn't take long before his cock began to stiffen up again, and soon it was so swollen that I could hardly get it in my mouth.

"I made a real show of licking it and biting it. I ran my teeth all the way down to his balls like I was eating sweet corn. I crammed both of his balls into my mouth until I practically gagged. I was a little drunk, I'll admit it. But I was much more intoxicated by what I was doing, sucking Theo's cock in front of all these people, and sucking it so well that all the men had hard-ons and all the girls were jealous. Some of them came real close to watch what I was doing. One of the girls took hold of Theo's cock and rubbed it against my lips like a giant lipstick. Everybody was getting so turned-on it was unbelievable. Well, me included.

"I flipped up the back of my dress with my left hand and pulled down my panties. They weren't very big panties, just like a little triangle of transparent black lace. Another girl helped me to pull them right down and gave them to me. They were all damp, of course, because I'd been sucking Theo's cock and that had made me wet myself. I wrapped them round the shaft of Theo's cock and used them to rub him, and at the same time I gave him such a licking and a sucking that everybody in the whole room was going wild. Three of my girlfriends held the cheeks of my bottom open, so that my cunt was exposed, and all of the guys started to finger me. I was too busy sucking Theo's cock to notice how many there were, but at one point three or four guys had their fingers in my cunt and my asshole, maybe more. Theo was so stiff that I knew he was just about to come, and with all those fingers inside me, I was just about to come, too.

"Theo gripped my shoulder hard. That was it. He was coming. And do you know something, for some reason, even though I'd sucked him out in front of so many people, I wanted his climax to be something personal, just between him and me. So when he came, I closed my mouth over his cock, and he shot his sperm right down my throat. I swallowed it and gave his cock one last suck, and that was it. Just at that moment, there were lights outside in the driveway, which was my friend's parents coming home, so the party broke up. But everybody was talking about it for months afterward, and every boy in the whole neighborhood asked me for a date.

"I wasn't any kind of an expert on oral sex. But I think I did it well because I enjoyed it. That was all it took. It's the same for a woman. If a man really enjoys licking your cunt, if he goes down on you like he wants to eat you and drink you and breathe you, if he wants to wash his face in your cunt juices and lick you all over, then it's fantastic. It turns you on, it gets rid of all of your tensions, it carries you away.

"Like, I think sex is all about forgetting everything except the person you love, shutting out all of your problems, and concentrating on *him* and nothing else."

Gillian's first act of oral sex may have been more exhibitionistic than most, but she's perfectly right when she talks about concentrating on your partner and nothing else. Women who are good at fellatio concentrate on the oral stimulation of their lover's penis to the exclusion of their own immediate desires. They don't think: *once I've sucked his cock for two or three minutes we can get on with normal lovemaking.* They kiss their partner's penis. They suck it. They lick it. They roll it against their cheeks and entwine it in their hair. They give it butterfly kisses with their eyelashes.

Women often seem to forget about their partner's genitals once they are no longer erect. They don't realize that men derive a considerable amount of pleasure from having their balls and their softened penises massaged and stroked and made a fuss of. If a man fails to achieve an instantaneous erection when a woman fondles his cock, the woman immediately takes this as an indication that he doesn't find her sexy any longer, or that he doesn't find her caresses exciting or stimulating. This couldn't be further from the truth. The sexually irresistible woman is the woman who knows that sometimes her partner may be tired, or stressed, and that he simply won't be able to achieve a full erection, just because she's squeezed his penis two or three times and tickled his testes. He will, however, greatly enjoy the intimacy of having his softened penis stroked, and his balls played with, particularly, if you don't make him feel that he *must* have a hard-on, and that he *must* make love to you.

Rheanna, twenty-five, a photographic processor from New York, New York, works very demanding hours—as does her boyfriend, Kevin. "I love sex, and I like oral sex the best. I love going down on Kevin and I love it when Kevin goes down on me. Sometimes he fills his mouth with ice water when I'm least expecting it, and squirts it up inside me, and that really makes me shiver. I love sucking him when he's hard, but I love it equally when he's soft, too. After we've been making love and he's lying on his back half asleep, I can take his cock and his balls into my mouth and gently suck them. They taste of *his* juices and *my* juices, all mingled together, and they're delicious. And, no, I don't expect him to have another erection. I'd probably be too tired to make love to him again even if he did. I just like the feel and the taste of his cock in my mouth, that's all. Do I have to make excuses?"

Charlene, twenty-nine, a graphic designer from Santa Cruz, California, recommends that you do even more than licking and sucking. "I like to decorate my lover's cock in all kinds of different ways. You remember Mellors, in *Lady Chatterley's Lover*, who wound daisies into her pubic hair? Well, I like to wind flowers into my lover's pubic hair, and I also like to suck his cock until it's stiff and then draw designs on it with a felt-tip pen. Sometimes I can make his cock look almost tribal, you know, with swirls and curves. Once I drew a shark's mouth on it. Another time I painted his balls with gold paint and made paper angel's wings that I stuck on either side of his cock. I do it for fun. But I also do it out of love. And he absolutely loves me stroking and caressing and painting his cock."

While we're on the subject of decorating your partner's penis, many women have written to say that if I'm in favor of women shaving off their pubic hair, why can't men do it, too? "I'd love to go down on my husband," said twenty-five-year-old Rosa, from San Diego, California. "The trouble is, he's so hairy! He has very thick pubic hair all around his cock, and his balls are hairy, too. Whenever I try to go down on him, I feel like I'm choking on hair."

These days, an increasing number of men are shaving or trimming their pubic hair, mainly because their partners prefer it. Dean, a twenty-eight-year-old physical training instructor from St. Petersburg, Florida, said, "It's all connected with bodybuilding and aerobics and the whole body-culture ethic. Most of the bodybuilders I know treat their bodies like sculpture, you know? So they have no body hair whatsoever. But ordinary guys who work out and look after their hair and their skin and their nails, they keep their pubic hair trimmed, too. They usually shave their balls so that they don't have any unsightly long hairs hanging down, and their girlfriends won't be deterred from sucking them. They like to keep a small, well-trimmed 'beard' of hair around their cock, so that they still look manly, but they keep their actual cock completely free of hair, so that their girlfriends can take the whole thing down their throat without any problems. I see naked men every single day of the week, and I have to say that men look better if they've paid a little bit of attention to keeping their pubic hair in shape. Me? I don't have any hair at all. My wife loves it that way. She doesn't have any, either. She says you don't know what it's like to be really naked until you've shaved off your pubic hair. When you make love it's just skin against skin."

Even women who have been involved in a long-term sexual relationship can still find their partner's sexual organs to be mysterious and complicated and rather alarming. But if you make a point of getting to know your lover's penis at close range—looking at it, touching it, caressing it, kissing it, sucking it—then you will soon begin to think of it as a sexual plaything, rather than some kind of threatening totem pole. You will find that you are far better sexually adjusted, far less anxious about sex, and you will be able to give your partner far more sexual pleasure. Just remember: ever since he was little, your partner has been playing with his penis. Now it's your turn.

Just one warning: don't expect that every time you play with his penis you're going to get a super-hard erection followed by instant lovemaking ... and try not to give him the impression that you do. All we're talking about here is an intimate, affectionate caress. It may lead to something, but it may lead to nothing at all, except a feeling that you love him, and that you want to be close to him, and sometimes a feeling like that is worth all the orgasms in the world.

The sexually irresistible woman:

- Wakes her partner up on Saturday mornings by sucking his penis.
- Opens his pajamas and fondles his penis while he's watching late-night TV.
- Cups her hand between his legs in the middle of a heavyweight cocktail party.
- Follows him to the bathroom and insists on holding his cock while he pisses.
- Masturbates him in the shower.
- Spends an evening giving him a shower, a hair treatment, a massage, and finishes up with the longest, slowest, most lascivious act of oral sex that he's ever had the pleasure to experience.

When you control your partner's penis, you control your whole sexual relationship. I'm not talking about being dominant, or withholding sex because you're angry with him, or offering him oral sex as some kind of reward for giving you something that you want, like a diamond necklace or a trip to Hawaii. I'm talking about the way in which you can control his timing, so that ninety percent of the time he gives you just the kind of sex you want whenever you want it. So many sexual relationships run into trouble because, most of the time, men can reach a climax with far less stimulation than women—leaving women aroused but unsatisfied. But once women take charge of their partner's penis, this problem is largely alleviated. Masters and Johnson were the first Western researchers to suggest that a woman could delay her partner's premature ejaculation with their famous "squeeze technique," but we've already seen how you can speed or delay your partner's climax without him even realizing what you're doing.

When you're in charge, you'll find it easier to achieve an orgasm more quickly. Deirdre, twenty-five, a systems analyst from Denver, Colorado, said, "I exercised my vaginal muscles with weights every day for four months, and every night I pleasured myself using a dildo. It took me a while, but I found all the right angles of penetration that really turned me on. If I'm sitting up, and the dildo presses against the front wall of my vagina, that stimulates me so much. And if I flex my muscles at the same time, kind of *ripple* them, if you know what I mean, I can bring myself to an orgasm within three or four minutes, sometimes less. I tried it with my boyfriend, David, and it worked even better with a real, live cock! I set up this rippling movement, which started my orgasm, and even David felt it. He said it was like having his cock massaged by three women at once. I had a wonderful orgasm, one of those wonderful spiritual ones when you feel like your whole mind is expanding all the way across the universe. And what made it even better was that David wasn't anywhere near to climaxing; his cock was still hard as a post, and right up inside me. So when he kept on thrusting and thrusting, I started to ripple my muscles again and I had another orgasm and then another and another. I swear I had four full orgasms before David finally climaxed inside of me. Of course *he* felt proud, because he'd satisfied me so much, and I certainly wasn't going to disillusion him, because it was *his* personality and *his* body and *his* cock that had turned me on. But at the same time I knew that it was *my* fitness and *my* self-knowledge that had made it possible for me to have so many orgasms."

The sexually irresistible woman recognizes that she can't leave all of the responsibility for sexual satisfaction in her partner's hands. No matter how brilliant and considerate a lover he is, she still has to develop her own sexual skills so that she can subtly adapt his lovemaking to suit her own particular needs. Oral sex is one of the best ways in which she can start this subtle adaptation, while at the same time fulfilling one of his most fervent fantasies.

Some women are still understandably hesitant about the business of swallowing (or not swallowing) their partner's sperm. Again, this is a matter for your choice alone. You may have consented to oral sex. You may even have initiated it. But that doesn't automatically imply that you're willing to swallow your partner's ejaculate. Some women adore it, and can't get enough of it. Anne, a twenty-one-year-old dental assistant from Surrey, in England, described in a British magazine how she had visited a sex club in Cologne, Germany, with her friend Carla. After an orgiastic evening with ten couples, Anne said, "My body was coated with sweat which was licked off by three of the girls, who sucked my cunt and my bum, my armpits and my breasts." Then Vera, the club hostess, asked her if she was willing to try "a special drink."

"She fetched a glass and gave it to one of the girls who started jerking off the prick of one of the men. The other couples did the same, rubbing the stiff cocks. One by one the men came, their semen being collected in the glass, which ended up almost full. Vera handed it to me and I smelled its contents: thick, warm sperm. I raised the glass to my lips and let the sexy fluid run over my tongue before swallowing. I drained the last drops, savoring the taste, my lips dripping with sperm. Everybody applauded me."

While this was probably an exaggeration (even ten men would find it difficult to fill an entire glass with semen) there isn't any doubt that many women acquire a taste for sperm and thoroughly enjoy swallowing it—not least for the obvious pleasure that it gives their partners. Gilda, twenty-eight, a hotel receptionist from Miami, Florida, said that she had always avoided oral sex in case any of her partners climaxed in her mouth. "But one evening I dated George, who was this totally gorgeous fitness instructor. He took me back to his apartment and we made love every which way. He was so strong . . . he actually picked me up and made love to me standing up. Then he went down on me and started to lick my pussy. His tongue was strong, too. It swirled around and around and I was in heaven. He poked it right into my pussy and I practically saw stars. Of course his cock was right over my face, and I couldn't resist taking hold of it and kissing it, just the tip of it, which was all that I could reach. But he lowered his hips down a little and I was able to lick it and take it into my mouth. His cock was huge and his balls were so tight and wrinkled they were like enormous walnuts. He slowly started to fuck me in the mouth, pushing his cock deeper and deeper. Usually it doesn't take much to make me gag. You know, a spoon in my mouth, anything. But when George pushed his cock into my mouth I didn't feel like gagging at all. All I wanted was more of it.

"At the same time he kept on licking me and licking me and I was so close to having an orgasm that every muscle in my whole body was locked up. George suddenly tensed and I knew that he was going to climax. He tried to take his cock out of my mouth but I wouldn't let him. I wanted him to come in my mouth. I could feel his cock going pump-pump-pump—and my mouth filled up with this warm slimy stuff that tasted like—I don't know what it tasted like. Sperm, I guess. That's all I can say. I let it slide down my throat and then I licked my lips. It didn't taste like anything I'd ever tasted before but I liked it. In fact I sucked his cock to get out the last few drops."

As we've seen before, it doesn't matter if you don't like the taste and texture of semen. You can always give your partner a sexy spectacle by directing his ejaculating penis toward your face or your breasts or your stomach.

A serious word of warning: don't have unprotected oral sex with a man of whose medical, social, and sexual history you aren't one hundred percent sure, and don't taste or swallow his semen. You can give your partner very arousing oral sex even when he's wearing a condom, although you'll probably need to give him some vigorous hand rubbing to bring him to a climax. As twenty-two-year-old Jayne said, "I don't mind giving head now that you can buy fruit-flavored condoms. It doesn't spoil it too much, wearing a rubber. I like it when they climax, and the little bulb on the end suddenly fills up with sperm. You can bobble it from side to side with your tongue."

It's surprising how many manuals and lovers' guides forget about the very basics of making love, kissing and caressing. It's also surprising how many couples forget to kiss and caress each other before they make love. Slow, tender kisses and slow, tender caresses not only show how much you feel for your partner, but prepare you physically and emotionally for eventual sexual intercourse. Next time you kiss your partner, make sure that you take control. Prevent him from putting his tongue in your mouth (by closing your lips) and instead put your tongue inside of his. Hold the sides of his head while you're kissing him, in the same way that a man would hold a woman. Kiss him all over his cheeks and his chin. Lick his closed eyes with the tip of your tongue. Bite gently at his earlobes.

Men are very aroused by love bites, especially around the neck and the nipples, but *don't* do it where it's going to show over his collar line. There's nothing quite so tasteless as a man turning up for a business meeting with a huge hickey on his neck. And don't do it at all if you're "borrowing" him from his wife or another long-term partner. It's not up to you to make the decision to tell them that he's been playing the field.

The same goes for scratches. Kelly, twenty-one, a telephone salesperson from Flint, Michigan, had a brief affair with her thirty-two-year-old boss. "One day we both went crazy. We spent nearly two days in a hotel room, doing nothing but fucking and sucking and living off room service. Lyle loved me digging my fingernails into the cheeks of his ass, and one time I dug them in so deep that their was blood all over the sheets. I even dug my fingernails into his asshole, until it hurt him so much that he shouted out loud. He had the greatest climax ever, but his ass looked as if it had been mauled by a tiger. He managed to hide the scratches from his wife for about ten days, but one morning he was lying asleep facedown with his ass showing, and she woke up first and saw the marks I'd made. They nearly divorced."

Running your fingers through your partner's hair and caressing his scalp will gently arouse him, as will trailing your fingertips down the sensitive sides of his naked body, around the tops of his hips, and down the outsides of his thighs. You can turn him on with all kinds of little teases, like butterfly kisses (fluttering your eyelashes against his cheeks and his nipples and the head of his erect penis). Small, sharp bites to his nipples may excite him, but be careful not to bite too hard, or stimulation can easily become irritation. You can nip the flesh of his upper thigh, too, and even take the skin of his scrotum between your teeth and drag it from one side to the other like a dog worrying a bone. Scrotum-biting looks much more ferocious than it really is—but again, be careful that you don't bite too hard and cause a wound.

All the time that you're kissing and caressing your partner, remember that you can arouse him with very much more than your hands. Your nipples can brush against him, your feet can slide down the inside of his calves, your hair can trail across his penis, your pubic hair can tickle his thighs.

Wendy, twenty-three, who works in a restaurant in Grand Rapids, Michigan, said, "I have very long brunette hair and my boyfriend loves it when I wrap it around his cock and masturbate him with it. Once when he was lying on his back half asleep I wriggled my head into position between his legs, face upward, and started to kiss his balls and his asshole from underneath. Then I had an idea and started to push my hair up his asshole with my finger, almost all of it. You can bet that woke him up! I kept on kissing his balls and masturbating his cock with my hand, and when I felt his sperm dropping onto my face I slowly drew my hair out. He said that gave him a feeling like silk sliding out of his ass."

You can devise your own caresses according to your physique and your sexual inclinations. Many large-breasted women enjoy pressing their breasts tight together so that their partner can make love to their cleavage. It's also possible for a man to make love to the cheeks of a woman's bottom without actually penetrating her anus.

Janice, twenty-four, a very lithe, slim girl from Providence, Rhode Island, said that her "usually staid" husband loved it when she smothered herself all over with baby oil and massaged him with her own naked body.

But never forget the simple, lingering kiss—even when you've been married for twenty years. When you kiss a man and you mean it, it shows. Even if you never attempt any of the sexual variations described in this book, never forget what you can tell your partner with a kiss. It may be old-fashioned, but it's always irresistible.

After oral sex, the act that men fantasize about the most is anal sex, which we've already talked about in some detail. The gentlest anal caress, licking around the anus, is called anilingus, and if your partner is in a calm and receptive mood, you can arouse him almost to the point of climax with the tip of your tongue alone. You can insert one or more fingers in his anus (making sure that your fingernails are well-trimmed) or you can slide your entire hand into it.

If you want to try "fist fucking," as it's known, you will have to treat your partner with very great care and make sure that you thoroughly lubricate your hand with K-Y. Never force your hand into his anus; let him open himself out so that you can slide your fingers in. And if he complains that it hurts, immediately but smoothly take your hand out again.

Vicki, a thirty-two-year-old secretary from Dayton, Ohio, discovered fist fucking almost by accident. "I never knew that you could actually put your whole hand up a man's asshole. I never knew that a man would actually *like* it. But last year I was having a thing with this guy I met at work, Martin. Tall, dark, and very handsome. We got talking while he was waiting to see my boss and since it was practically the end of the day he asked me if I wanted to have a drink with him.

"I wasn't attached or anything, so I said why not, and that's how it started. He took me out to dinner a couple of times. He brought me flowers. He was always very polite. One thing led to another, and one night he took me home and we listened to some Alanis Morrisette and made love.

"I thought he was a pretty good lover. Better than my ex-husband, Joe, anyway. But there was something he nearly always did when he made love to me that I wasn't used to. I didn't say I didn't like it . . . I just wasn't used to it. When he was near to climaxing, he pushed his finger into my asshole—sometimes just the tip, sometimes all the way in. I got used to it after a while and began to enjoy it. In fact I enjoyed it so much that I thought that I'd do it to *him*.

"He was lying on his side on the bed one night.

We'd been making love and we were both all sticky. I dipped my finger into my vagina and then I traced a wet line all the way down between the cheeks of his ass until I reached his asshole. I circled my finger around and around it for a while, and then I prodded my finger right in. His asshole was quite tight, but my finger went in easily. I kind of stirred my finger around and he shifted a little. I reached around him with my other hand and I could feel that his cock was rising, quite quickly. I rubbed his cock and stirred my finger around some more. Then I managed to slip in a second finger, which meant that I could waggle them up and down inside his asshole. His cock was seriously hard by now, and I kept on rubbing. I tried to force a third finger into his asshole, but he said, no, use this, and next to the pillow he found the lubricant we'd been using. He rubbed it all over my hand, and then he opened his legs really wide. It was easy to push three fingers inside. Then I managed to fold my hand and push in a fourth finger, and my thumb, too. Martin gasped out loud. I'll never forget that gasp. His cock was immense, and I kept on beating at it and beating at it. I pushed my whole hand into his asshole, stretching his asshole wide, and then it closed around my wrist. I could wriggle my fingers inside his ass, but his muscles were very tight and that was about all I could do. I wriggled my fingers and rubbed at his cock and suddenly he climaxed, without any warning at all. There was loads of sperm, but it didn't shoot out of his cock, it *poured*, like somebody emptying a jugful of cream all over my hand. I carefully pulled out my hand and he held me in his arms and kissed me. He didn't say a word. I mean, what can you say after something like that?"

The reason for the flowing nature of Martin's climax

was probably due to the fact that Vicki was stimulating his prostate gland, which is responsible for producing the basic fluid of which semen is composed. The prostate can be felt by inserting your finger into your partner's anus. It is a soft, tissuey mass a few inches inside the front wall of the rectum, and you can stimulate it without going to the extreme of forcing your whole hand into his bottom.

At first, he may not find the sensation of having his prostate massaged very agreeable. It can be sensitive, even painful. But if you persevere you will discover he begins to enjoy it, and eventually sperm will start to flow out of his penis, whether he has an erection or not.

What about *him* inserting his fist into *you*? A famous German sex video series, *Maximum Perversum*, has a feature entitled *Tango in the Dark*, in which a handsome blonde man in a tuxedo rolls up his sleeve and pushes his entire fist into the anus of a statuesque girl in a black basque and black frilly stockings. But unless you're very experienced in anal sex, your partner's hand will probably be too big for you to accept inside your anus, and it's wiser for you not to risk any tearing of anal tissues by attempting it. His finger will give you all the anal stimulation you need—or maybe he'd like to make you a gift of a thin anal dildo or a vibrating latex "butt plug."

When you practice anal sex, always remember that the rectum contains virulent bacteria and that even if your hands don't *look* dirty you must always wash them thoroughly before touching your vulva. Similarly, make sure that your partner washes his penis before attempting vaginal sex, even with a condom.

Another sexual variation that turns men on is bondage—tying you up and having their wicked way with you while you're completely helpless. It turns on a great many women, too. There are varying degrees of bondage, from simply fastening your wrists and your ankles to the head of the bed with scarves or neckties, all the way through to using steel handcuffs, restricting corsets, arm restraints, and leather helmets that leave you blind and deaf and unable to speak.

Absolutely unshakable rule number one: never practice any kind of bondage with a man you can't implicitly trust. No ifs or buts. And don't forget the other rules, either. Bondage games must always be played out with the full consent of both partners. You must never fasten anything around your neck, or restrict your breathing in any way. Don't use knots that are difficult to untie. Never leave a tied-up person alone. Never play bondage games unless you're one hundred percent sober. And last of all, agree beforehand on an "instant release" signal that is always honored without any hesitation.

It's interesting to find that many of the men who enjoy bondage games are comparatively quiet and passive in their everyday sexual behavior, even shy. Bondage games give them the opportunity to act out a dominant role in the bedroom according to formalized rules, and to exercise a power over women that doesn't come naturally to them.

Sandy, a twenty-six-year-old blonde who works in an art gallery in St. Louis, Missouri, had her first taste of bondage with Robert, whom she met quite casually at a launch party. "Robert attracted me because he was so quiet and reserved compared with everybody else there. He was very good-looking and I saw quite a few women go up to him and talk to him, but his quietness seemed to put them off.

"I went up to him myself and asked him if he liked

the exhibition. He said he did. Then I asked him if he'd like me to freshen his drink and get him something to eat, and he said sure, he'd like that. You wouldn't think it, but these quiet guys like people to run around after them. Most of the time people say, 'Hi, how's it going?' and then ignore them. If you offer to do something for them, no matter what it is, it makes them feel special, that you're interested in them, and that starts to bring them out.

"It was hard work at first. But the more I talked to Robert the more I liked him. He was bright, he was funny, but he was just incredibly unassertive. Mind you, I made up for both of us. I gave him the full Sandy seduction treatment. Deep, interested looks; standing up close with lots of touching and brushing. Asking him to hold my drink for me while I took a telephone call, so he was making himself useful to me and he knew that I was coming back. No—I didn't adjust his necktie. It was straight already. But I would have, had it needed adjusting. There's something about adjusting men's neckties that practically makes them weak in the knees.

"By the end of the evening, I had Robert eating out of my hand. He invited me to go to a concert that weekend, Rachmaninov. I said sure, okay, and I felt quite pleased with myself. But the very next evening he came into the gallery just before we closed, carrying a bunch of roses. He asked me if I would have dinner with him. He said he couldn't wait until the weekend to see me again; he'd had me on his mind all night. Well, what can you say to an unassertive man who plucks up enough courage to do that?

"We had a great Italian meal and then he drove me home. He kissed me, and I kissed him back, but that was as far as it went—for that night, anyway. But all the same we knew that we liked each other. If I had any qualms about Robert, I guess it was the way in which he always asked me what *I* wanted to do, and what *I* wanted to drink, rather than make up his own mind. I'm not saying I don't like consideration and courtesy in a guy; I do. But I do like a man to take charge, especially when it comes to ordering wine and deciding where we're going to go to eat.

"He came over on Saturday around seven o'clock to take me to the concert. He was wearing a tux and he looked absolutely great. I was wearing my slinkiest black evening dress with spaghetti straps. I think some kind of chemistry had been working between us since that Wednesday night, because as soon as he stepped in the door he took me in his arms and kissed me, and I kissed him, too; and before we knew it we were locked in this embrace like two long-lost lovers.

"Robert said, 'I have a confession to make.' And I thought, 'Uh-oh, here we go, he's married. I might have guessed.' But then he said, 'I hate Rachmaninov.' And I looked up into those blue, blue eyes of his, and I said, 'What a coincidence. I hate Rachmaninov, too.'

"That must have been the most subtle invitation to bed that any man ever had. We walked across my apartment strewing our clothes behind us like we were acting in some romantic movie. By the time we reached the bedroom, Robert was naked and I was struggling to pull my dress over my head. We got to the bed and my arms were still up above my head, tangled in my dress. I tried to pull it off but Robert said, 'No . . . I like you like that.' He lifted me onto the bed and climbed on top of me. He may have looked like one of your shy, soft guys but he was very strong and fit, and he had a terrific flat stomach. His cock stood out like the handle of a bullwhip, all veiny and knotted. I would have done anything to touch it but my hands were still tangled up in my dress.

"I tried to struggle free but Robert kissed me and then he ran his hands down my body and suddenly struggling didn't seem so very important. He cupped each of my breasts in both hands in turn, and kissed my nipples, and then he ran his tongue all the way down my stomach and licked my navel. All the time he was giving me these beautiful compliments, I can't even remember what they all were, but things like, 'Your skin . . . I never came across skin as soft as this before.'

"It was strange. Nobody had ever made love to me like this before. But I could see that Robert was very turned on by the fact that I was semihelpless. He gently opened my legs so that he could look at me. My cunt was shaved completely bare, and I could tell that turned him on, too. He opened up my cunt lips with his fingers and looked at it, then he looked up at me and there was this smile on his face like you wouldn't believe. He said, 'You're too amazing for words,' and I knew that he meant it because in the sunlight that was coming through the window I could see a drop of juice glistening on the end of his cock.

"'Condoms in the drawer,' I told him, but he'd brought his own. I hadn't noticed him scattering them on the bed when he came in. He held his cock in his hand and rolled on this shell-pink condom. Then he nestled the head of his cock between the lips of my cunt. He leaned forward and kissed me again, and I wondered when the hell he was going to put his cock right in. My cunt was absolutely burning for it. He kissed my breasts and nipped at my nipples with his teeth and *still* he didn't put himself right in. If I'd had my hands free I would have grabbed hold of his butt and pulled him into me, but of course I couldn't, and that was the whole point of what he was doing. He was making me wait. He was exercising his power over me. I wanted to push his cock right inside me, but he wouldn't, and there was nothing I could do about it.

"I began to get aroused and panicky at the same time. I squeezed my cunt muscles around the head of his cock, as if I could suck it right up into me. It was a funny thing, but all of that rhythmical squeezing really turned me on, especially since I could just feel the tip of his cock inside me.

"He said, 'I want you so much,' and that was when he actually pushed his cock right inside me, until I felt his balls up against the cheeks of my bottom. His cock was immensely hard and very long—longer than my ex-husband's cock, longer than any cock I'd ever had. It was so long that when it went right inside me it made me spasm, but all I wanted was more.

"He took it out again and kept it out, and I could feel the juice between my legs. 'For God's sake, fuck me,' I told him, but he still wouldn't put it back in. 'Robert, if you don't fuck me—' And still he didn't put it back in. It was then that I understood what he wanted. This was a bondage game, a power game. 'Please, Robert, pretty please. I'm begging you, Robert, fuck me.'

"He fucked me. He really fucked me. He took hold of my hips and lifted them up off the bed and rammed that big, long cock into my cunt until I was gasping and panting and screaming at him not to stop. He turned me over onto my stomach and fucked my cunt from behind, squeezing and massaging my breasts while he did it. Then he lay me on my back and fucked me from the side, with his fingers playing on my clitoris. He started to fuck me with deeper and deeper strokes and I could feel that he was close to coming.

Just *thinking* about it gave me a sudden orgasm, one of those almost unexpected ones, and when I started to climax he climaxed, too, so that was pretty good—a simultaneous orgasm our very first time together.

"Afterward I went to the kitchen and poured us both a glass of sparkling wine. I had bought it for *after* the concert, believe it or not, as a way of seducing him! We lay on the bed together and kissed and touched each other and it wasn't long before we made love again, and then again.

"I said to him, 'Are you into bondage at all . . . the way you wanted me to keep my arms all tied up in my dress?' He was kind of reticent about that, but I said, 'Come on, you loved it when I was all tangled up and helpless . . . that meant you could do what you wanted with me, and I couldn't do anything about it.' He said, 'Didn't *you* like it?' And of course I realized that I had—maybe more than I had cared to admit to myself.

"I've always been so confident and self-sufficient that it was quite exciting to find that I was suddenly helpless, and that a man could do with my body whatever he wanted, and I wouldn't be able to stop him. It was only a game. I wasn't really helpless, and I know that Robert would have stopped if I had asked him to. But all the same there was this really erotic sense of being *possessed*, if you know what I mean."

Sandy went on to have more bondage games with Robert. "His favorite was to tie my wrists to the bed rails with scarves, and sometimes he'd knot my hair around one of the bed rails, too, so that I couldn't move my head. He tied my ankles to the foot of the bed so that my legs were apart. Occasionally he used a blindfold so that I couldn't see what he was doing.

"He was always incredibly gentle with me. He was never rough. But that didn't mean that what he did wasn't very, very sexy. He used to massage my breasts with different oils and make me guess what fragrance they were. Sometimes he would stroke the inside of my thighs with a big soft artist's brush, and just run it lightly down the slit of my cunt. Other times he used to 'draw' on my naked body with ice cubes. Or else he'd chill his tongue with an ice cube and lick my clitoris . . . not touching me anywhere else at all. If you've never been given an orgasm by a cold tongue tip, you haven't lived, believe me.

After a year, Robert's company sent him to the West Coast. He asked Sandy to come with him. He even asked her to marry him, but after a lot of heart-searching she declined. "He gave me a year of affection and romance and some of the most incredible sexual experiences I've ever had in my life," she said. "But in the end I knew that it wasn't really love. In the end I knew that I needed a man who could assert himself without having to resort to playing games. All the same, he taught me things that nobody else could have taught me, and I fully intend to use them when I meet another man that I want to go to bed with."

Sandy got along so well with Robert because she paid attention to what he said and did, and very quickly realized what kind of a lover he could be. She thought of *his* pleasure first and her own second, but because of that she was given, in her own words, "some totally mind-blowing orgasms." The type of bondage that she enjoyed with Robert wasn't at all extreme, and many couples get pleasure from occasional tying-up sessions—whether it's the man who ties up the woman, or the woman who ties up the man.

Just as nonassertive types like Robert are aroused and satisfied by making love to a helpless woman, so many dominant and assertive men derive sexual stimulation from being rendered helpless themselves. Many of the men who regularly visit prostitutes in search of bondage and domination are men in authority—industrialists, police officers, judges, bankers. In her "torture chamber" in The Hague, in Holland, the dominatrix Monique von Cleef used to administer enemas to some of the most powerful men in the country and then hang them upside down by their heels, their heads buckled up in leather masks. Others would have to wear penis cages with spikes inside them and all kinds of leather cock leashes and ball-separating straps and rubber underwear. Monique would sit them down on a little three-legged milking stool to tell them a nursery story. The stool sported an immense wooden dildo in the middle of the seat, which the client would have to insert into his anus.

This, of course, was fairly heavy-duty sadomasochism, and unless you have a very keen interest in bondage and restraint, my advice is not to get involved in it, even if you meet a very beguiling man who wants you to. There's no harm at all in enlivening your sex life with occasional excursions into slave-and-mistress-style games, but you will find that men and women who are deeply into S&M practices tend to be unable to achieve sexual satisfaction without all of their rituals and their paraphernalia, and while there is nothing morally wrong in what they do, heavy sadomasochism is not the stuff that everyday long-lasting sexual relationships are made of.

As thirty-two-year-old Francesca said, "I loved Dick dearly, but I couldn't love his helmets and his leather gear and his rubber stockings and all that stuff. I couldn't stand the *smell* of it, to begin with. It frightened me, if you want to know the truth. He always wanted me to dress up in red rubber stockings and ridiculously high heels and tight rubber hoods that covered my eyes. Whenever we made love he called me Miss Scarlett and begged me to tell him how bad he'd been and how disgusting he was and how I was going to whip him. In the end I'd had enough. I loved him, but I think he loved Miss Scarlett, not me. He's probably found some other poor woman to play Miss Scarlett by now."

However, less obsessional sadomasochism can be harmless and highly stimulating. Marie, twenty-three, a singer from Los Angeles, California, said that her long-term partner, an influential record producer called Bill, occasionally enjoyed "a little light punishment." "I found out about it very gradually, but I'm glad that I did, you know? Because apart from being a turn-on for me, Bill finds it a way of relaxing and unwinding and getting rid of all his tension. Like, five days a week he's responsible for everything, right? His business, his staff, his press agents, his artists. When he comes back to me on the weekend he doesn't want to be responsible for anything. Just for a while, anyhow. So we disconnect all the telephones and play."

Marie said that she discovered Bill's enjoyment of sexual punishment after they returned home from a party. "We were arguing, because Bill had been monopolizing this one woman all night, and I wonder why. She only had larger breasts than all the other women in the room put together, and a dress that looked as if it had been sprayed onto her naked body. Bill had already undressed by the time I was finished in the bathroom, and when I came through to the bedroom he was lying facedown on the bed, naked. He kept on denying that he'd spent too much time with this girl, and I kept shouting back at him that he'd made a fool out of me in front of everybody. I got so crazy with him I took my slipper and I slapped his bare ass with it, real hard, so that it left a bright red mark.

"I expected him to be mad. But instead he stayed where he was, with his face buried in the pillow, and he didn't say anything at all. I slapped his ass again, and then again, and then again, until his cheeks were flaming red. Then suddenly he rolled over and took hold of me and laid me down on the bed. There were tears in his eyes but his cock was standing up hard. He said, 'You're right. I deserved that. Are you going to forgive me?'

"I was still angry. I said, 'No, I'm not going to forgive you . . . making a spectacle out of me like that.' All he did was turn facedown again. I hesitated for a moment, I'll admit, but I was beginning to guess what it was he wanted. I slippered his ass again and again, maybe five or six times. He rolled over again and this time his cock was softer. I looked at the bed and I suddenly saw why. All that slippering had made him have a climax all over the sheet.

"Now, whenever he's had a stressful week and he comes home shouting and tense, I make him take off all of his clothes, even in the living room, and I slipper his ass until he climaxes. Sometimes I make him hold on to the top of the doorframe and I slipper him standing up. That's great, because when he climaxes I can see him spurting sperm all over the floor.

"We hardly ever made love when he came home on the weekends because he was wound up too tight, like a clock spring, and all he could think about was work. But these days things are really different. He says that I spank all of the tensions out of him. I know for sure that when we make love afterward it's almost always wonderful. That's because his mind's on me, instead of his work."

Celestine, twenty-six, from Chicago, Illinois, who's black, tall, and very eye-catching, occasionally plays an erotic game with her partner, Paul, who's white. "We don't play it very often, but sometimes we'll start thinking about it during the week and by the time the weekend comes, we're all turned on and really looking forward to it. It doesn't have anything to do with our normal relationship, which is pretty average, I guess, and pretty romantic. Maybe we feel that we need to go beyond the boundaries now and then.

"Most of the time, I'm the mistress and he's the slave. I wear nothing at all except for this fetish costume made of black leather straps that leaves my breasts bare. It's crotchless, too, except that it has three silver chains across the hole, so that my pussy kind of bulges out between the chains. I wear these black leather thigh boots with six-inch high heels, and I always carry a whip. Paul has to call me 'mistress' and he has to ask my permission any time he wants to do anything at all. He's usually naked, too, except for this black leather metal-studded ring that I make him wear around his cock and balls. It has a ring in it that I can snap a dog leash on to and I lead him around after me. We bought all of this fetish stuff out of a mail-order catalog and we'll probably buy some more. I liked the look of a cock restraint that has straps all the way up it." She smiled when she said this, as if she couldn't wait to try it out.

"I make Paul wear leather wrist cuffs all the time. I make him cook for me and if he makes a mess or he doesn't hurry I tug his cock ring and whip his ass. He's not allowed to use a fork to eat with and if he makes a mess I pull his cock ring under the table. After the meal he has to lick the plates completely clean before he puts them into the dishwasher, no matter what's on them. I make him go outside the apartment and empty the trash even though there's a risk that somebody might see him. That's part of the thrill! Once I shut him outside, completely naked except for his cock ring, and he had to beg to get back in again.

"After we've eaten I'll give him some chores to do, like licking my shoes clean or scrubbing the kitchen floor on his hands and knees. I like him doing that because I can whip his ass if he misses a spot. At bedtime he'll run my bath for me and fill the bathroom with lighted candles. Before I have a bath I'll go to the toilet, and if he's been good I'll allow him to lick my pussy clean. He washes me in the bath and he's allowed to soap my breasts and my nipples and wash between my legs. Afterward he has to dry me with a towel.

"Only when I'm lying ready on the bed, powdered and perfumed, will I finally take off his cock ring. Even then I might not take it off for maybe ten or twenty minutes, and lie there with my legs wide apart, masturbating myself in front of him, tugging out my clitoris, sticking fingers into my pussy and licking them and *daring* him to touch me. He can look, you see, but he isn't allowed to touch me until I say so. At last when I'm feeling ready, I say, 'Come on, then,' and he'll lie back on the bed so that I can ease myself down on top of him. I fuck him then the way I want to fuck him, very slow and very easy. But his cock's always very hard, and I know that he's aching to shoot his sperm up into me. I tease him with the whip, flicking his cheeks. I say things like, 'You want to shoot your sperm up into me, don't you? Well, I don't know if I'm going to let you. Maybe I'm going to find some other man and let him shoot his sperm up into me, and what will you do then? Then sometimes I take the whip handle and I poke it into his asshole, and twist it around, and all the time the rules of the game are that he does what I tell him to do, because I'm the mistress and he's the slave.

"He tries to make sure that I have an orgasm first, because if I don't I always punish him, biting his nipples and whipping his balls. He's really learned how to hold himself back, because he knows that if he doesn't he's going to have his balls and his bottom and his asshole whipped, and that *hurts*. And when I've had an orgasm, and he's had his climax, too, I always make him crawl down between my legs and lick all of his sperm out of my pussy. He has to kiss me with his mouth filled with sperm so that I can taste it, too. It's only when he's finished kissing me, and I've licked the last taste of sperm out of his mouth, that I grant him his freedom. He isn't a slave anymore, he's my lover, and we're back on equal terms."

Celestine and Paul weren't serious sadomasochists. Like many couples, they enjoyed a sexual vacation now and again, acting out an erotic fantasy that excited both of them. They felt like playing out their game of mistress and slave only very occasionally, when the mood took them. Occasionally Paul took the role of the dominant partner, and Celestine was equally excited by that, although Paul said that he felt he preferred to play the part of the slave. "I think there's something in every man's psychology that wants to be humiliated. Whenever I'm Celestine's slave, I think of myself as X—a man with no name and no identity, who exists only to be humiliated by a dominant woman."

For her part, Celestine understood that there are times when a man can be highly aroused by being humiliated or hurt by a woman—just as there are times when he might want to excite himself by doing something dangerous, like parachuting or skiing or whitewater rafting. The human psyche is very complicated and often contradictory, but the sexually irresistible woman understands that the man in her life might have widely differing sexual needs and fantasies. One time he might feel like a cuddly evening making love on a blanket in front of a crackling log fire. Other times he might feel like a wet-sex session, with he and his partner spraying urine over each other in a ceramic-tiled bathroom.

Practically all men respond to a greater or lesser extent to sadomasochistic stimuli. Even the straightest man can be turned on by having his back scratched or his nipples bitten. That's why men are irresistibly drawn to women who behave as if they might be able to dominate them and tease them and control them. Try being a tigress with your lover tonight, and see what a difference it makes.

Apart from oral sex and anal sex and bondage there are many erotic scenarios that men rarely include on their list of top ten turn-ons, but that you can use to excite him far more than he ever imagined possible. Once you have brought any one of these fantasies alive for him, he'll find it very, very difficult to find a woman more sexually irresistible than you.

CHAPTER EIGHT

Sexually Irresistible . . .
That's You

One of the things I suggested you do during your All-Day Self-Pleasuring Session was to list your special fantasies and secret desires. I've asked men to do the same thing, and it's fascinating to compare what they consider to be the top ten turn-ons with the sexual scenarios that excite women the most. Men are much more aroused by variations in *technique* (oral sex, anal sex, mutual masturbation, making pornographic home videos, vibrators and other sex toys, three-in-a-bed, partner-swapping, fingering and fisting, wet sex) than they are in *how* and *where* lovemaking takes place.

Women on the other hand talk about making love in a field of flowers, or having hurried sex in an elevator. They talk about meeting their partners at the office wearing nothing but a raincoat. They list the places that turn them on, and what they'd like to be wearing. "I can't think of anything sexier than making love in the backseat of a big black limousine, dressed in nothing but a black garter belt and black silk stockings," said Mara, twenty-one, an advertising executive from Philadelphia, Pennsylvania. And Sonya, twenty-eight, from Bangor, Maine, said, "My fantasy has always been to make love totally naked on a heap of furs in front of a fire, while it's snowing outside and the windows are all frosted up."

Gillian, a fifty-five-year-old senior executive for a New York catering company, said, "Would you believe it, I've never made love in a four-poster bed. I'd adore that. Maybe me and two young men, with the drapes drawn tight. I'd wear a red basque and red stockings to go with my pubic hair, because that's red, too—natural red! And these two young men would compliment me on my breasts because my breasts are very big, and they'd kneel next to me and rub their cocks all over my nipples. Then I'd suck both of their cocks at once, a big mouthful, and afterward they'd both fuck me at the same time, until we were all exhausted. You see? I only have to *mention* four-poster bed and I get carried away."

It's interesting that women's erotic tastes vary very little because of age. Middle-aged women like Gillian have very similar fantasies to girls of nineteen and twenty, and just as intense. One of the most fascinating examples of this was the fantasy that forty-one-year-old Gaby, who worked as a tour guide in San Diego, California, shared with her nineteen-year-old daughter, Katherine. Gaby was a highlighted blonde, with a figure that had won her beauty contests when she was younger. ("They even asked me to pose for *Playboy* when I was seventeen, but my father refused to allow it. . . . That was one of the great regrets of my life; I'd have *loved* to have posed for *Playboy*.) Gaby was divorced from Katherine's father. ("He was a workaholic . . . I still love him, but there were too many separations, too many late nights. . . . We didn't make love for a whole seven months, and I'm afraid to say that I need my sex.") Katherine had very similar looks to her mother, except that she had her father's brown eyes. Katherine was at music college, with an ambition to write musicals like *Cats* and *The Phantom of the Opera*.

Gaby and Katherine planned on having Sunday brunch at Cardiff-by-the-Sea, but they had to wait for a table and so they spent a half hour on the beach. "There was a guy surfing, not too far away from us," Gaby recalls. "He was very tall, very muscular, very handsome indeed. He had short blonde hair and terrific teeth. Twenty-two years old, as we later found out. He wore these tight yellow shorts that showed that he was *very* well endowed, and Katherine and I both agreed that he was a ten . . . or even an eleven.

"We watched him surfing. He was very powerful and graceful. As we watched him we started talking about sex—you know, the way you do when you're watching a half-naked man with great muscles and bulging shorts. I told Katherine for the first time that one of the reasons her father and I had split up was because he didn't give me enough sex. Heaven knows, I didn't have a boyfriend and I wasn't getting any sex at all at the time, but if I'm going to have no sex at all I'd rather live alone than go through the frustration of lying next to a snoring man with a floppy cock.

"Katherine said that she was very attracted to a boy at her college, but he already had a steady girlfriend and so she didn't think she had much of a chance. She had talked to him and flirted with him, and in the end he had jokingly said, 'You like me, my girlfriend likes me. We'll have to sleep three in a bed.' "

He didn't really mean it, of course, but the idea had kind of stuck in Katherine's mind.

Katherine herself said, "I kept having fantasies about what it would be like for two women to take one man to bed . . . all the things they could do to him, and all the things they could do with each other. I'm not a lesbian, but I do think that some women are very sexually attractive, and I've often wondered what it would be like to kiss another woman and touch another woman's breasts. This fantasy about having three in a bed wouldn't leave me alone, and I embroidered it more and more. I used to think about it late at night, and masturbate before I went to sleep."

Gaby was surprised at her daughter's fantasy. It hadn't shocked her, because sexually she was a very liberal-minded woman. But it was almost exactly the same as one of the strongest of her own sexual fantasies. When she was in her late teens, she had walked into a bedroom at a party at her friend's house, thinking it was the bathroom. She had surprised her friend with another girl. Both of them had their skirts up around their waists and their blouses open, and they were jointing fellating the college's football captain.

"That made such an impression on me—partly because I was so embarrassed, partly because I was very sexually innocent in those days, and I was shocked. But I kept thinking about it afterward and I began to realize that it had made such an impression on me because it turned me on—because I would have liked to have joined in."

Mother and daughter didn't consciously plan to fulfill their fantasy with the surfer on the beach. But after a while he came to sit close to them, and Katherine got into a conversation with him. His name was Joe and he was an English student at UC San Diego. He had a girlfriend but she had gone to spend the weekend with her parents in Santa Barbara.

Gaby said, "I suddenly realized that both Katherine and I were flirting with him, both in our different ways. He started off shy, not saying much, but we managed to draw him out and make him laugh. In the end I said that we were going for lunch at the Blue Dolphin and would he like to join us. He said he wouldn't be able to afford it, but I said that I'd pay. I said that we were long overdue for some male company. Joe went back to his place to change, and Katherine and I talked about him and agreed what a great guy he was, but even then I don't think we clearly had in mind what we were going to do. Life's like that sometimes, isn't it? It's like you put your conscience on hold, and allow yourself to be swept along. Otherwise you'd probably never do anything daring or exciting or interesting."

Katherine said that brunch was "wonderful." "We drank about four mimosas each. I wouldn't say that we were drunk, but by the time the meal ended we were definitely feeling very friendly. Mom asked Joe back to her apartment in La Jolla for another drink, and Joe said, sure, why not, it beat the hell out of surfing. Even then—yes, I'd agree—we still weren't consciously planning to take Joe to bed. And we sure weren't planning on going to bed with each other. I mean—mother and daughter—no way. But everything that happened, happened naturally. Nobody was forced to do anything, and nobody had to be persuaded."

Gaby drove them all back to her third-floor apartment overlooking La Jolla Bay. "We were all laughing and everything was very informal. I had three bottles of Napa Valley Brut left in the icebox—they were left over from a party I'd given the previous month. I poured out three glasses, and then I went into the bedroom to change out of my blouse and my jeans and take a shower. You always get so sandy and hot on the beach; you feel like a broiled lobster.

"When I came back, Katherine and Joe were out on the deck, talking and laughing together. I was wearing nothing but my yellow satin bathrobe. I said to Joe, 'You're going to make me jealous, flirting with my daughter like that.' I looked him right in the eye and I guess there was something in the way I looked at him that *emboldened* him, you know? It was like a challenge. Because he put his arm around my waist and he kissed me, right on the lips, and smiled; and then he said, 'There . . . you don't feel jealous now, do you?'

"Katherine said, 'Maybe Mom doesn't feel jealous, but *I* do.' So Joe turned around and gave her a kiss, too. It started off as fun, but you could see that they were strongly attracted to each other, because this one fun kiss went on and on. I said, 'Now I *am* jealous.' I held his face in my hands and kissed him, pushing my tongue into his mouth and licking his teeth and his tongue. Maybe it was all those mimosas, I don't know, but I put my hand down and grasped his crotch, and his cock was so hard that it was practically breaking out of his jeans. He had a button fly, instead of a zipper, and I plucked his buttons open one by one. Underneath he was wearing the whitest boxer shorts I'd ever seen, and they were so full of cock that it was unbelievable. I hadn't had a man's cock in so long I guess you could say that I went a little bit crazy. But I pulled down his shorts and his cock came out. It was big and purple and the hole in the end was gaping at me. I heard Katherine saying, '*Mom* . . .' like she couldn't believe what I was doing, but I went down on my knees in front of him and I took his cock into my mouth and I sucked it, and it was heaven. It felt like heaven, and it tasted like heaven. You can't tell me that there's anything in the whole world that tastes like a man's cock when he's in heat. It tastes like sex and piss and heaven."

Katherine said, "I couldn't believe what Mom was doing. Joe and me were really getting it on when she started playacting that she was jealous and that she wanted a kiss, too. I didn't mind the first kiss, but when she started pushing her tongue down his throat and groping his crotch, right in front of me, I just couldn't believe my eyes. Then she opened his jeans and took out his cock. You never saw such a big cock. He wasn't circumcised, but his foreskin had rolled back so that the head of his cock was completely bare, and it was dark, like plum color, and he was literally dripping this transparent juice out of the end of it, a long sticky string that went right down to the rug. And Mom knelt down and opened her lips and took the whole of his cock right into her mouth . . . I mean he was so big that she had to stretch her mouth wide open.

"I guess I had several options open to me right then. I mean this was my mom, right? I could have left her and Joe to get on with it, and come back on hour later, trying to pretend that nothing had happened. Or I could have stamped my feet and gone into a tantrum, and called my mom a whore. But why was she a whore? She wasn't married, after all. She might have been my mom, but she was still a woman with her own sexual feelings and her own desires. And if Joe liked her, what was the problem?

"The funny thing was, I *still* wasn't thinking about our fantasy of two women making love to one man. I'd forgotten it, in the heat of the moment. But I knew that when my mom made love to Joe, I didn't want to be left out. Why should *she* have all the fun, just because she was older? I pulled down Joe's jeans at the back, and then I pulled down his shorts, baring his ass. He turned around and said, 'Hey!' but it wasn't very convincing because Mom had his cock in her mouth, almost up to the balls. There was coral lipstick all around it, like a rash. I said, 'Hey, yourself!' and I kissed him, and groped his ass. He had the most beautiful ass. It was white, because he hadn't been sunbathing naked, but it was so tight and round and muscular. I dug my nails into the crack between his cheeks, and poked his asshole with my fingernails, and I didn't hear him complaining, not once.

"With my left hand, I reached around and took hold of his cock. It was still buried in Mom's mouth, but I ran my fingers all around her lips and all around his cock. Mom said, '*Mmmm . . .*' and sucked his cock even more deeply. I stroked her face and her hair. Then I pulled Joe's jeans and shorts right down, and fondled his balls. I love men's balls. I love the way they go all soft and relaxed after they've finished making love, but I love them best when they're tight and wrinkled. I think what I like about them most is that they're so sensitive. A man can have muscles like Tarzan and tattoos all over him and a really bad attitude, but he's still got balls—sensitive, tender balls. Like, when you take a man's balls into your mouth you've got him, haven't you? He wants you to do it, he likes it, but it would only take one really hard bite and you'd have him begging for mercy.

"I said, 'Come on, Mom, let's do this inside.' Like, when we're out on the deck, people can see us. None of us said a word. We went through the living room, into the bedroom, and immediately Mom loosened her robe and let it fall to the floor, so that she was naked. I hadn't seen her naked for years, and I couldn't believe what a fantastic figure she had. She was tanned all over . . . even in her armpits . . . this lovely golden honey color. Her breasts were as big as mine. They were softer, but they were still firm, with enormous nipples. Her stomach was rounded, but what can you expect after three children? Her cunt was completely hairless, and it was beautiful, like a flower, you know? And her bottom was firm, too, because she'd been exercising. She had a pattern of moles on her back which she always used to tell me was just like the constellation Cassiopeia. I suppose I should have been embarrassed, or shocked. I guess most people are, when they see their parents naked. But here was a totally beautiful woman . . . a woman who looked like me, and talked like me, and felt like me, and I loved her.

"Joe sat on the bed and took off his jeans and his T-shirt. I don't think he understood what was happening any more than we did. If one of us had said, 'Stop! What the hell are we doing here?' I think we would have stopped. But I think all three of us wanted it to happen, and I think Mom and me wanted it to happen even more than Joe did.

"I took off my blouse and unfastened my bra, and then I dropped my skirt. I was wearing a black lace G-string but I didn't take it off. I climbed onto the bed next to Joe and ran my fingernails across his chest and all around his shoulders and said, 'I'll bet when you woke up this morning you never would have believed this was going to happen to you.' And he said, 'I don't believe it's happening to me now.'

"I knelt beside him and kissed his mouth and his neck and his shoulders and his chest. I didn't love him. I think back about him now, and I don't feel any sense of loss. But he was a great guy, a beautiful personality, and he had such a wonderful body; and if men can treat women like a sex object, why can't women do the same with men? You know what my Mom and I did that day? We took this beautiful suntanned guy with a great big penis and we fucked him, we used him, and why not?"

Gaby said, "I climbed onto the bed naked and knelt on Joe's chest and arms, pinning him down, kissing him. I loved kissing him because he was so young and smooth. I kissed his neck and his chest and his nipples. Then I sat astride his face, with my cunt only inches over his mouth. He tried to lick it but he couldn't reach it. It was so juicy that it was literally dripping onto his chin. He tried sticking his tongue out as far as it would go, but I still wouldn't let him reach it. Then Katherine put her hand underneath Joe's head and lifted it up. He stuck out his tongue and licked my clitoris, and then he ran his tongue all the way down between the cheeks of my ass.

"I looked at Katherine and she looked at me. She was my daughter but we were both women and we both had strong desires. I ran my hand into her hair and stroked her cheek, and Joe caught the mood between us because he turned his head and kissed Katherine, and then he kissed my cunt, and then he kissed Katherine again, with his lips all wet from my cunt juice. I don't know whether I felt this was right or wrong. All I felt was an overwhelming love for my daughter, and a great sexual excitement, like being so hungry that you can't wait to start shoveling food into your face.

"Joe licked my cunt again and again, and I lowered myself down on his face so that he could suck my cunt lips. He rolled up his tongue and pushed it right up inside my cunt. I hadn't been so wet for years. I was so turned on that my juice was pouring out of the sides of his mouth and down his neck. Katherine licked it up, and kissed his neck, and gave him two or three love bites. I don't think either of us cared what his regular girlfriend was going to think about them.

"I sat right down on Joe's mouth and he gave me the most comprehensive cunt-sucking that I've ever had in my life. He was tugging my clitoris into his mouth and flicking it with his tongue. He was poking his tongue into my pee hole, which nobody had ever done before. He was drinking the juice that poured out of my cunt and licking my asshole.

"What I didn't realize was that Katherine had gone down the bed and was kissing and sucking Joe's cock."

Katherine said, "I don't think I've ever been so sexually excited in my life, not before or since. I watched Joe licking Mom's cunt for a few moments. The way his tongue rolled around her clitoris was such a turn-on . . . and to watch it close-up! Then he pulled her cunt wide apart with his fingers and stuck the very tip of his tongue into the hole she pisses from. She doesn't remember it but she moaned when he did that. I ran my hand over Joe's stomach. It was so taut and hairy. Then I took hold of his cock and gripped it tight. He was almost as wet as my mother . . . he had juice running down his cock and into his pubic hair. So how could I resist it? I slid down the bed and took the head of his cock into my mouth and gave him a deep, deep sucking. I played with his balls and tugged at his pubic hair, but most of all I took that great big cock of his into my mouth as far as I could, until I actually started making choking noises.

"I sucked Joe's cock and almost swallowed his balls. Then Mom came further down the bed, too, and it was obvious that Joe wanted to fuck her. I said, 'Come on,

Mom—not without a condom.' She had plenty of condoms in the top drawer of her dressing table, and I went to get one for her. I tore open the foil and put the condom in my mouth . . . then I leaned over Joe's cock and rolled the rubber right down his shaft, using my lips. My mom was watching me, and I'll bet that's the first time in history that a daughter has put a condom on a man's cock so that he could fuck her mother.

"Mom climbed on top of Joe and opened her legs up wide. I parted her cunt with my fingers, so that Joe could push his cock in more easily, but while I was touching her, I thought, this is incredible, this is my mother's cunt. I was actually *born* out of this cunt, and here I am touching it and feeling it. Joe was trying to push himself in but I wouldn't let him, not yet, because I wanted to slip my fingers up inside Mom's cunt and feel what it was like. It was warm and it was slippery and it was so sexy, and yet it was comforting, too. Sometimes I wonder what it would be like to touch my father's cock, the cock I came out of. It's just incredible, to think that this was how you were created, out of sex, out of two people urgently wanting to fuck each other.

"Anyhow, Joe urgently wanted to fuck Mom, so I took my fingers out of her cunt and I held his cock and guided it into her. She sat down on it and let out this deep sigh, like this was something that she'd been looking forward to for months. She rode up and down on him a few times, and both of them were gasping and moaning, and there was no way that I was going to let them fuck themselves into an ecstasy without me joining in. I put my head down between my mom's thighs and licked Joe's balls. They were all tight and hard, and slippery with my mom's cunt juice. I licked the lips of my mom's cunt and Joe's cock, where they joined. Then I licked my mom's asshole, and she made a sound like nothing you've ever heard. I stretched her asshole even wider with my fingers and pushed the tip of my tongue into it, and I could feel her *shudder*, you know, like a goose had walked over her grave.

"I'd been tugging my thong up between my legs, and my cunt was so juicy that it was nothing but a wet string. I pulled it off and I was just about to toss it away when I thought of something else I could do. I think I must have read it in one of your books. I pushed my wet thong up my mom's asshole while she and Joe were fucking, until there was nothing showing but a loop of black elastic. Joe was fucking her harder and harder. She was shouting at him, 'Fuck me! Fuck me!' She orgasmed, and when she orgasmed I slowly pulled my thong out of her asshole, wet black scratchy lace, and I think that just about blew her mind."

Gaby said, "Both of us lost all of our inhibitions. It was the best time we'd ever had together. We kissed each other, cuddled each other, mother and daughter, but lovers, too. Our breasts brushed together, we kissed each other's nipples, we touched each other between the legs. For a while Joe could hardly get a look in. But then his cock started to rise up again, and I said to Katherine, lie back and suck him, and then I'll see what I can do for you.

"Katherine lay back on the pillow and took hold of Joe's cock. To start with, he wasn't totally hard, but then she kissed his glans and clutched hold of his balls and his cock began to stiffen up again. I took hold of his cock, too, and opened Katherine's mouth with my fingers, and steered his cock right into it. I kissed the side of her mouth, and Joe's cock, too. She started to suck him and I could hear those little squeaky noises in her mouth as she practically swallowed him alive.

"It was then that I went down on Katherine's cunt. I hadn't ever done that to a woman before, let alone my own daughter. But she was an adult; she was so beautiful. Her cunt was covered in this fine blonde fur, like mine used to be before I had it waxed. Because she was so much younger than me she was even juicier than me, and when I first licked her between the legs I thought she might have wet the bed. But it wasn't that, it was all juice.

"I closed my eyes and tried to imagine that this was *my* cunt. I licked her clitoris just the way that I liked it licked, very quickly, from side to side. I sucked her pee hole, because that's something that sends shudders through me. Then I opened her vagina as wide as I possibly could and plunged my whole face into it, licking her hole, smothering her juices all over my cheeks and my eyelashes, breathing her in, that sweet delicious taste of a young woman's cunt, my daughter's cunt.

"I rolled another condom onto Joe's cock and he made love to Katherine while I lay beside them. I was tired now, but I ran my fingers down Joe's back and around his ass and cupped his balls. I stroked Katherine's breasts and pulled at her nipples and tickled her down between her legs. It took Joe a long time to climax, but when he did, Katherine came, too, and all three of us lay on the bed, sweaty and exhausted and smelling of sex. I think we all knew that this would never happen again—couldn't—because we'd broken all of the rules that you can possibly imagine. Katherine and I haven't spoken about it until now, and I don't think that either of us would ever tell anybody else what we did. But the way I see it, there are times when you can break the rules and discover what you are and who you are, and experience feelings that nobody else in the world is ever going to experience, and so long as you don't hurt anybody or cause them any kind of psychological damage, then who's to say what's right and what's wrong? All I know is that for a few minutes in my lifetime I had my face in my own daughter's cunt, and during those few minutes I was in ecstasy.

"She and I had the same fantasy, and she and I fulfilled it together. Do you think that it would have been any more moral if she had fucked Joe with a friend of hers, instead of me? I don't know. That's a question that nobody can answer, isn't it?"

Personally, I was much more interested in what Joe had thought about his experience. Had he considered that the fulfillment of Gaby and Katherine's fantasy had made them sexually irresistible or not? It took me some time to find him, but when I did, he was very frank about what had happened. "They attracted me. They also frightened me. Can you believe that? Most of the girls I'd dated before had been very much younger. I fucked them, and they said, 'Oh, Joe, you're terrific, I want to marry you.' Then they would follow me around for the next six weeks looking at me with these Bambi eyes. But these two—Gaby and Katherine—forget it. They were women. I didn't realize that they were mother and daughter until halfway through, when Katherine suddenly said, 'I love you, Mom,' or something like that, because Gaby had such a great figure and she looked so young. But, you know, when you look around, older women *do* look younger these days, and what's the problem with being older if you can fuck like Gaby can fuck?

"They frightened me but it was a good fear. It was an exciting fear. It kind of drew me toward them, you know? They were confident, they knew what they wanted out of sex, and sometimes I think it makes a change for the man to feel like he's being hunted, instead of the other way around."

Hadn't he thought of seeing them again?

"I don't think so. Individually, maybe. But which one would I choose? All the same, they taught me a whole lot. They taught me to look at women in a different way. These days I don't look at forty-year-old women and think, 'Don't bother, you're past it.' Older women fuck as good as younger women, and I think what happened to me with Gaby and Katherine is living testimony to that."

The lesson is: don't be hesitant about involving the man in your life in *your* fantasies. Chances are your erotic ideas are much more exciting than his. You can always include what he wants to do in your fantasies, after all. Maid Marian can allow Robin Hood to have anal intercourse with her, as a reward for rescuing her from Nottingham Castle. The slave girl in the Eastern market can always give her new owner a seriously good evening of oral sex.

Some of the most irresistible fantasies that women have come up with are:

The Bridal Fantasy—Jolene, twenty-four, from Houston, Texas, had a white wedding. On her wedding anniversary, she dressed up in her bridal veil, and carried a bouquet of flowers. But apart from that, all she wore was a white satin peephole bra, a white lace garter belt, and white stockings. No panties, but a fragrant white rose in her vagina. When her husband, Rick, came home, she announced that it was their second honeymoon—and Rick agreed. "She looked so sexy, but at the same time she looked so pure and virginal, she knocked me out. And the rose was a great touch— like I was deflowering her all over again."

The Adam and Eve Fantasy—Sue, nineteen, from

Napa, California, invited Calvin, twenty-two, for a picnic. In her own words, she had *adored* Calvin from the moment she had first set eyes on him, although he had been studying hard at law school and didn't appear to be very interested in her. "When we arrived at the picnic site, in the woods, I took off all of my clothes. All of them. I said that I always ate my picnics in the nude. I lit a campfire naked. I laid out all the food naked. I sat on the bench with my legs apart. If only he'd known how scared I was! But it all worked out. After about twenty minutes he took off *his* clothes, too; and about five minutes after that we were lying on a blanket, making love.

The Dangerous-Sex Fantasy—Vivian, twenty-seven, from Charleston, South Carolina, had been dating her boss at the insurance corporation where she worked but wasn't at all sure that he intended to continue their relationship. He was estranged from his wife but still saw her regularly, and Vivian believed that they still had sex—"out of need, out of guilt, who knows?" That was why she arrived at work one day with no panties under a very short skirt. She went into his office, lifted her skirt to expose herself, and zipped open his pants. She produced a condom, rolled it onto his rising cock, and sat on his lap. "He didn't even have time to tell his secretary to hold his calls. I fucked him. *I* fucked *him*. I did it again, too. I followed him into the executive washroom and fucked him up against the wall. I think he's scared of me, to tell you the truth. But who do you think he fantasizes about when he goes home at night? His wife, or me?"

The Baby Doll Fantasy—Trixie, nineteen, from Richmond, Virginia, had a serious crush on her music tutor, John, twenty-five. "The trouble was, he always talked to me as if I was a child. He was always so adult and pompous. He gave me the feeling that God would give him credits in heaven because he hadn't touched me. But there were only six years between us, and I was sure that I could seduce him, if I tried. Accordingly, Trixie played up the very thing she believed to be John's weakness. She guessed that the reason he treated her so remotely was because he was afraid of his own feelings toward a very pretty young girl. She was, in fact, exceptionally pretty, and she emphasized her looks by wearing lipstick and eye makeup every time she went for a music lesson, deeply scooped T-shirts that showed off her considerable cleavage, and minuscule skirts, with no panties. "I behaved like a baby doll, too. Leaning right over him so that my breasts pressed against his arm, saying, 'Please John, will you show me those notes again?' I was playing the part of his fantasy girl, and I laid it on so thick that in the end he *had* to give up. He asked me out, and five hours later we were in bed together."

You probably have a fantasy of your own. Whatever it is, don't hide it, don't be embarrassed by it—share it with the man you want to attract. The four women who tried my All-Day Self-Pleasuring Session came out full of confidence in their own sexuality, and each of them managed to fulfill their fantasies.

Ella, the dental nurse, who had fantasies about making love in the great outdoors, met an accountant—nothing like the football jocks she had always attracted in the past. He was a quiet and reflective man, but he deeply appreciated all of Ella's personal qualities, not just her sexuality but her love of nature and the joy she felt when she listened to music and poetry. He took her on a weekend vacation and made love to her "naked—both of us—on the warmest of nights, under a full, full moon."

Barbara, the cosmetician, who had fantasies of masochism, met two different men—one at a party, and one at a local tennis club. The man she met at the party had been going through a difficult divorce, for which he blamed himself. Barbara "punished" him for what he had done by making him wear her underwear to work and hitting his buttocks with a hairbrush whenever he forgot to phone her or turned up late. The man she met at the tennis club gave *her* the treatment she thought she needed by tugging down her panties whenever he felt like it and fucking her—leaving her sperm-filled but unsatisfied. Between the two of them she was beginning to find a balance, and she was confident that—before too long—she would be able to start a "normal" relationship. Normal? "You know—no pain, no guilt, no punishment, just loving."

Linda, the magazine editor, found that the All-Day Self-Pleasuring Session had freed her of guilt about her interest in younger men. "So I'm older and they're younger. So what?" She formed a relationship with a twenty-six-year-old lawyer and said that she was "blissfully happy."

Nancy, the bank executive who had been worried about her appearance and her weight, met the owner of a construction company—"rugged, virile, handsome if you think that boulders are handsome, and rich." For his part, her new beau thought that Nancy was "absolutely the sexiest woman in the world, bar none . . . you should see her underwear . . . you should see her in bed . . . she's like Vesuvius."

I hope that in reading this book you've discovered (if you've ever doubted it) that you're capable of being the sexiest woman that you've ever known. You may have found some of the personal accounts in this book shocking, but then everybody has their own different view of sex and their own different levels of tolerance. As I've repeatedly said, you never have to take part in any sex act that disturbs or upsets you. Sex should always be pleasurable and fulfilling and fun.

At a time when so many fashionable manuals are counseling you to be guarded and reserved, I'm saying exactly the opposite. Life is too fast and too short to play games with people's feelings, and that particularly counts for men who have genuinely shown some interest in getting to know you better.

The new millennium is a time for openness and warmth. It certainly isn't the time to be returning to the pinched social mannerisms of the 1900s. Women have already discovered their sexual strength, and now they can exercise that strength to find themselves the men they want, the relationships they want, the future they want.

You're sexy already. Go out and be irresistibly sexy.